Principles of Chest Roentgenology

A PROGRAMED TEXT

Benjamin Felson, M.D.

UNIVERSITY OF CINCINNATI COLLEGE OF MEDICINE
AND CINCINNATI GENERAL HOSPITAL

Aaron S. Weinstein, M. D.

UNIVERSITY OF CINCINNATI COLLEGE OF MEDICINE
AND CINCINNATI VETERANS ADMINISTRATION HOSPITAL

and Harold B. Spitz, M. D.

UNIVERSITY OF CINCINNATI COLLEGE OF MEDICINE
AND CINCINNATI GENERAL HOSPITAL

W. B. Saunders Company · Philadelphia and London

W. B. Saunders Company: West Washington Square
Philadelphia, PA 19105

1 St. Anne's Road
Eastbourne, East Sussex BN21 3UN, England

1 Goldthorne Avenue
Toronto, Ontario M8Z 5T9, Canada

Listed here is the latest translated edition of this book together
with the language of the translation and the publisher.

German (1st Edition) — Georg Thieme Verlag, Stuttgart, Germany

Japanese (1st Edition) — Hirokawa Publishing Co.,
Tokyo, Japan

Portuguese (1st Edition) — Atheneu
Editora, Sao Paulo, Brazil

Italian (1st Edition) — Piccin Editore, Padova,
Italy

Principles of Chest Roentgenology   SBN 0-7216-3605-5

Print No.:   25

To Virginia, Shirley, and Judy

INTRODUCTION

You are about to embark on what we hope will be a novel and rewarding experience. But first we'd better tell you something about the format in which you will be working. *Programed Instruction*, spelled with one or two *ms*, depending on the *avant-garde* spirit of the writers, stems from the Socratic method of advancing by easy stages from the simple to the more complex, guided by student response. It embodies a set of teaching concepts which include bits of information (in the form of "frames"), repetition, active student participation, and reinforcement by providing immediate answers.

The broad application and enthusiastic acceptance of programed learning by business, industry, government, and undergraduate education have been widely discussed. Yet its employment in medicine has been, to date, quite limited. Few medical programs are presently available and none deals primarily with the subject matter presented here.

Many advantages have been claimed for programed learning by its proponents. Our own experience is based on the presentation of most of the material in this book alternately to matched groups of medical students, the opposing group receiving the same information by illustrated lecture. Results of early and late examinations on the subject matter, evaluated by computer, and unsigned responses to a questionnaire for student reaction to this form of instruction were found to support some of these claims.

Each student worked at his own pace, obviously a very important advantage of the method. Long-term retention was slightly better with programed instruction. The top students performed well with either method, while the less proficient ones performed significantly better with the programs. The role that enthusiasm for *any* new teaching technique played in the improved performance could not be determined. However, one group of students who had had previous experience with programed instruction still seemed to favor the method.

We concluded early that it would be easier to train ourselves to program than to teach a programer the required amount of radiology. However, the preparation and testing of the programs proved to be a very time-consuming labor, which in the future we would like to delegate to someone else. Perhaps our greatest difficulty was to strike the proper balance between oversimplification and overcomplification, either of which seemed to discourage the students.

The programs were repeatedly tested on individual medical students and radiology residents, as well as in the classroom. One edition after another was prepared and tested until finally an acceptable version materialized. All the programs were then unified and field-tested in our own and several other medical colleges. Edited once more, the final result is in your hands.

An unexpected dividend accrued from the project. The lecturers competing with the program have taken a closer look at their own methods of teaching and have been stimulated to greater preparation and more dynamic presentation. This attitude of competition, while commendable, is really unnecessary since programed instruction is intended to assist the teacher, not replace him. It is supposed to free the teacher from repetitious pedantry and give him the time to clarify, emphasize, expand, and stimulate. These high-sounding aims have actually been achieved in other fields, so why not in medicine?

Programed learning has been linked almost inextricably with "teaching machines," which in our view are non-essential mechanical or electrical gadgets that often simplify the presentation and facilitate the response, but may in themselves be distractive. Some machines even prevent peeking ahead at the answers, which is not only frustrating and unfair, but downright insulting.

All the preceding discussion notwithstanding, our main purpose in this book is to teach some of the fundamentals of chest roentgenology to non-radiologists. Nearly every medical student and physician frequently finds himself face to face with a chest roentgenogram. Observing his discomfiture from a discreet distance, it seems obvious to us that he is attempting to interpret complex shadows without an adequate understanding of the basic concepts, like a one-eyed man trying to stereoscope. Of course, he can and does consult with the roentgenologist but, in the interest of his patient, he should have some knowledge of the roentgen approach. To gain this understanding he must, as with any other aspect of medicine, be grounded in the principles involved.

This program, then, aims to provide a background to chest roentgen interpretation simply and with a minimum expenditure of time. Much of the material emanates from a more conventional text also developed at the University of Cincinnati College of Medicine.* If the reader desires additional references, the bibliography in that book should help provide them.

Many individuals contributed to this effort. This is a new milieu not only for the authors but also for the publisher. The members of the W. B. Saunders Company staff deserve much credit for their enthusiastic approach to this new frontier. They have consulted with us almost from the beginning, going far

*Felson, B.: Chest Roentgenology. W. B. Saunders Company, Philadelphia, 1973.

beyond usual bounds to participate in the actual preparation of programs and subsidizing part of the cost. Deans Stanley E. Dorst, now emeritus, and Clifford G. Grulee, Jr., of our medical college, provided significant financial support and followed the project with deep interest. A host of medical students and radiology residents served as cooperative experimental subjects, and their strong reactions lent meaning to our work. Drs. Alvin A. Torf and John P. Christie, then medical students, were particularly helpful in this regard. Drs. Harold J. Schneider and Jerome F. Wiot were of inestimable assistance in the testing of the programs, and Drs. Theodore D. Sterling and Seymour V. Pollack not only supplied the computer analyses but also helped us construct some of the examinations. Mr. Richard L. Clark and Mrs. Ruth R. Friedman provided assistance with the photographs and diagrams. The scope of the secretarial effort was enormous but was handled efficiently and graciously, along with their many other duties, by the department secretaries, Claire P. Bittner, Mary Ellen Meyer, Sophie Travis, and Virginia R. Hagans.

Benjamin Felson
Aaron S. Weinstein
Harold B. Spitz

Cincinnati, Ohio

INSTRUCTIONS

Most of the numbered "frames" on the left-hand side of each page require a response. The questions have been intentionally designed in most instances to help you make the *correct* response — the answer is made clear by the frame itself or you have learned it in earlier frames. A single blank means you are to fill in just one word. When there are two blanks, fill in two words. When you find a blank preceded by a double asterisk (**), you should use as many words as you need to complete the statement.

In those frames which offer multiple choices, merely circle the one or more which you believe correct. Occasionally we have granted you respite by providing a frame in which no response is required. (Actually we had an answer prepared, but couldn't think of the appropriate question: just the reverse of the psychiatry professor who gave the same examination every year — but changed the answers.)

The answer to each frame will be found on the right-hand side of the page, and appropriately numbered. Use the "mask" in the back of the book to hide the answer to the frame you are studying. It is not essential that your answers be in words identical to ours, so long as the meaning is the same. If you miss an answer, re-read the frame so that you will be better prepared for what is to come.

At the end of each chapter is a review section summarizing the more important information and concepts you have just learned, or should have. Don't skip it. In the Quiz after the last chapter, a group of selected chest roentgenograms are shown to permit you to apply your new knowledge and to test your grasp of the subject matter. If you don't do well, blame us.

We prefer that you write your answers in ink so that your friends will have to buy their own copies. It's O.K. to cheat by looking at the answers first — it's your money and your time. Since concentrated attention is required, we suggest that you set a time limit, an hour at most, for consecutive study.

We trust you will not be disturbed by our zany attempts at humor and by the general informality of our program. These reflect our attempts to make the learning process pleasant and relaxing.

Have fun.

TABLE OF CONTENTS

Chapter 1

TECHNIQUES OF EXAMINATION

A basic understanding of the various types of chest roentgen examination is essential for every practicing physician. It is important that he know what information the various views and techniques can provide. The appropriate choice of a particular examination can expedite the work-up of the patient and thus facilitate a more rapid and accurate diagnosis.

1

Let's start with the standard frontal view of the chest, the posteroanterior <u>teleoroentgenogram</u> or, in oral shorthand, the PA teleo. The term *posteroanterior* refers to the direction of the x-ray beam, which in this instance traverses the patient from _____ to _____ .

posterior

anterior

2

This routine frontal view, taken with the patient upright and the x-ray tube aimed horizontally at a distance of 6 feet from the film, is what you get when you order a PA _____ view.

teleo

3   **3**

Why do we take the PA view at a distance of _____
feet?
To reduce magnification and enhance sharpness. See
for yourself:
   (a) Place your hand under a table lamp (bulb-type)
      and look at the shadow it casts on a piece of
      paper on the table.
   (b) Move the light closer to the hand and then
      farther away. As the lamp is moved away,   6 feet
      the shadow of the hand gets (smaller / larger)
      and (more / less) sharp.   (b) smaller
   (c) Now, keeping the lamp fixed, move your hand   more
      closer, then farther from the paper. The closer
      the hand is to the paper the (larger / smaller)   (c) smaller
      and (more / less) sharp is its shadow.   more

4   4

The anteroposterior (AP) view is usually made with
the patient supine. It is substituted for the PA view
with very sick patients, infants, or anyone else unable
to stand or sit. Obviously, in this instance the x-ray   anterior
beam passes through the patient from _____
to _____ .   posterior

This view is taken supine rather than prone because it is less awkward
for the sick patient, and the infant usually squawks less when he can
see what's happening.

5   5

Because of low ceilings and construction costs of
x-ray equipment (this is no joke!), AP views are
usually taken at a distance of about 36 inches and,
compared with the PA teleo, there is (greater / less)   greater
magnification and (greater / less) sharpness of the
images.   less

(If you missed this answer we suggest you repeat the experiment in
Frame 3.)

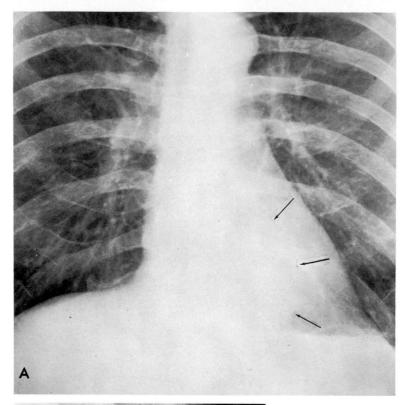

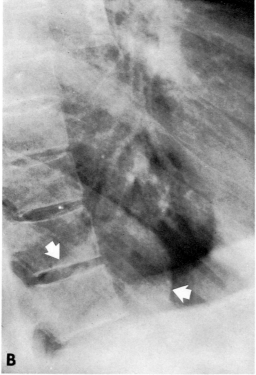

Figure 1–1

6

The upright is preferred to the supine view because
(1) it shows more of the lung, since the diaphragm
is lower; (2) it is quicker; and (3) it is easier to   sharper
attain 6-foot distance, so the images on the film are
_____ and less _____.   magnified

7

The other routine view is the lateral. The view in
which the left side of the chest is held against the
x-ray filmholder (cassette) is called a _____
_____ view.   left lateral

If we were consistent we would call it a right-left lateral, but "a foolish
consistency is the hobgoblin of little minds" (Emerson).

8

It is common for a lesion located behind the left
side of the heart or in the base of the lung to be
invisible on the PA view because the heart or diaphragm shadow hides it. The _____
view will generally show such a lesion, so we use it
routinely.   lateral

Figure 1-1, A, shows such a lesion (arrows), a cyst, which is barely
visible. We missed it in this view. The lateral view, Figure 1-1, B,
shows the lesion well (arrows).

9

To visualize a lesion in the left thorax, it is better
to get a (left / right) lateral view.   left

Remember the lamp experiment? The closer your hand was to the
paper, the clearer was its shadow.

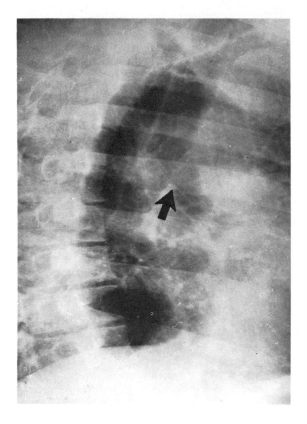

Figure 1–2

10

A fundamental rule of roentgenography: **Try to get
the lesion as close to the film as possible.** This
reduces _____ and enhances
_____ .

magnification

sharpness

11

Oblique views (often neglected by clinician and, alas,
roentgenologist) are used to localize lesions and project them free of overlying structures. For instance,
the tracheal bifurcation in Figure 1-2 (arrow) is best
seen in the _____ view.

oblique

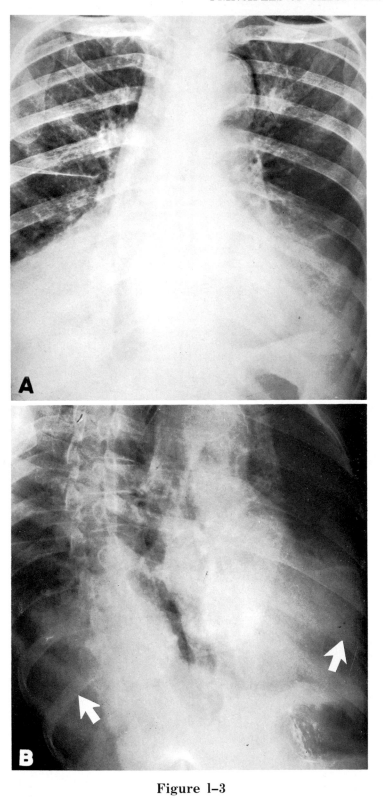

Figure 1–3

12

12

Figure 1-3, *A & B*, illustrates another reason for the oblique view. In *A*, bilateral involvement of the lower lungs by lymphoma is seen. In a lateral view it would be impossible, because of superimposition, to distinguish the right-sided disease from the left. The _____ view, in *B*, shows that the left lesion is anterior and the right is posterior (arrows).

oblique

The optimum degree of obliquity depends on the site of the lesion being studied and the information desired. It may have to be determined by fluoroscopy.

13

13

The direction of rotation for the oblique view is determined by the location of the lesion to be studied. The right oblique view is made with the front of the right chest touching the film. The left oblique is made with the _____ of the left chest touching the film.

front

You can figure out which oblique view is appropriate by imagining the lesion in your own chest and turning your body into the right and left oblique positions. When we're too tired to think we just take both obliques.

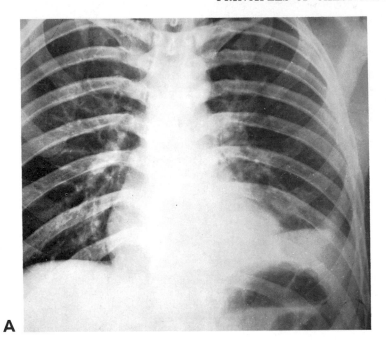

Figure 1–4

14   **14**

What other views are there? Free fluid in the pleural
cavity is affected by gravity. Fluid will gravitate
toward the diaphragm when the patient is _____,
toward the back when the patient is supine, and   upright
toward the lateral aspect of the dependent thorax
when the patient lies on his _____ .   side

In Figure 1-4, *A*, an upright film, what appears to be an elevated left
hemidiaphragm is really free pleural fluid which has gravitated to the
base of the left pleural sac. This is confirmed in Figure 1-4, *B*, made
with the patient lying on his left side. The fluid now lies against the
dependent left lateral thoracic wall.

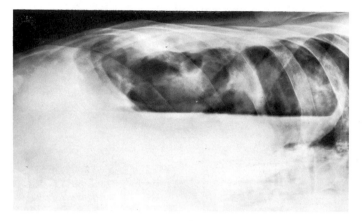

Figure 1–5

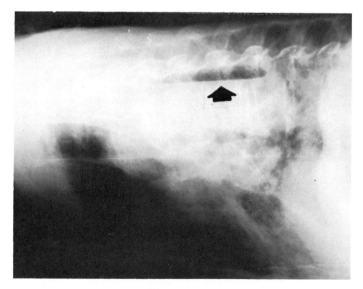

Figure 1–6

15   15

To demonstrate this gravitation of free pleural fluid, as well as to confirm air-fluid levels in the lung itself, a *decubitus* view is often used. It is made with the patient recumbent and the x-ray beam horizontal, i.e., parallel to the floor.

What do you think the word *decubitus* actually means?   lying down—We looked
**   it up in the dictionary.

Figure 1-5 is a film taken with the left side down, showing an air-fluid level in a huge right lower lobe abscess. See also Figure 1-4, *B*.

16   16

By convention, most x-ray technicians and roentgen-ologists define a decubitus view as one taken with the patient *lying on his side*. The x-ray beam, remember, is _____ to the floor.   parallel (horizontal)

PA teleo view: horizontal x-ray beam.
Decubitus view: horizontal x-ray beam.
AP recumbent view: vertical x-ray beam.

17   17

By our definition, a film made with the patient prone or supine, utilizing a _____ beam, could be called a prone or supine decubitus view. It seldom is, however; the usual term is *cross-table lateral view*.   horizontal

Figure 1-6 is a cross-table lateral view with the patient prone, showing an air-fluid level (arrow) within a large tumor.

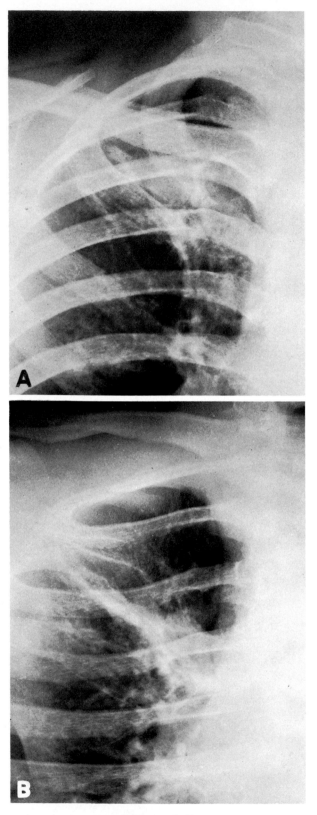

Figure 1–7

18

These inconsistencies have plagued physician and technician so much that sometimes the best way to get the view we want is to draw a picture or to say, for example, "Get me a cross-table view with the patient lying on his right side facing the tube." Incidentally, what should this particular view be called?

** _____

18

right lateral decubitus

19

Another important view is the *lordotic*, which is conventionally made in the upright AP position with the patient leaning backward at an angle of about 30 degrees from the vertical.

19

No answer required, thank you.

20

The lordotic position is obviously awkward for the patient. Someone finally made the momentous deduction that angling the x-ray tube instead of the patient would accomplish the same purpose. So now the patient faces the film as for a PA teleo and the tube is elevated and angled downward 45 degrees. With peculiar logic we still call this the _____ view.

20

lordotic

21

On the standard PA teleo film, the clavicles and upper ribs obscure much of the pulmonary apices. The lordotic view projects the apices below the clavicles and causes the ribs to project more horizontally, and thus provides a clearer view of the _____ of the lungs.

21

apices

In Figure 1-7, the lordotic view (*B*) shows the tuberculous lesion better than the routine view (*A*), because the shadows of the clavicle and ribs interfere less. Note the position of the right clavicle.

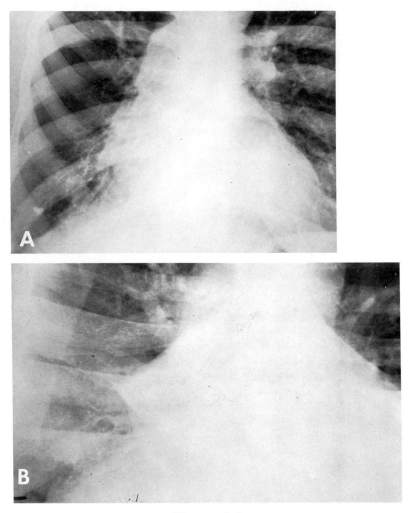

Figure 1-8

22

22

Two portions of the lung, the right middle lobe and the lingula, are relatively narrow in anteroposterior diameter and, in pneumonia or collapse, may cast little density. In the lordotic projection, the beam traverses the longest axis of the middle lobe and lingula so that, when diseased, they appear (more / less) radiopaque.

more

In Figure 1-8 the routine view (A) shows an ill-defined density obscuring the right heart border. In B, the lordotic view, a dense triangular shadow typical of right middle lobe collapse is seen.

23

23

To obtain a clearer view of the apices, or to better delineate disease in the right middle lobe or lingula, one should obtain a _____ view.

lordotic

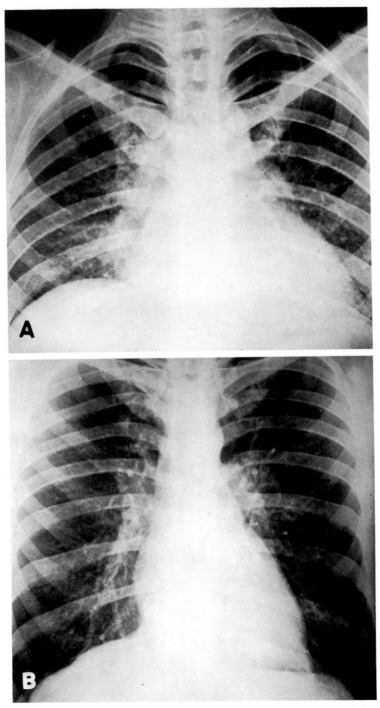

Figure 1–9

24   24

The normal chest film is, of course, made on inspiration. On expiration the lungs "cloud up" and the
heart appears (larger / smaller).   larger

> A favorite trick of radiologists is to test a student with a normal
> expiration film (Figure 1-9, *A*). A diagnosis of cardiac enlargement with
> congestive failure is usually made. *B* was made on inspiration a few
> moments later.

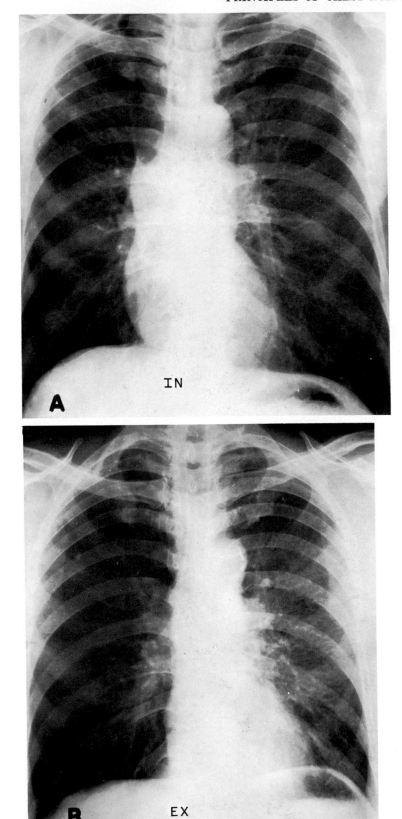

Figure 1–10

25

The expiratory film is very useful in detecting
unilateral obstructive emphysema. Since its air cannot
readily be expelled, the lung on the obstructed side
remains (expanded / contracted) and (radiolucent
/ clouded) on expiration.

25

expanded

radiolucent

Figure 1-10 shows carcinoma of the right main bronchus with obstructive emphysema. *A*, Inspiratory film; *B*, expiratory film. The right lung remains expanded.

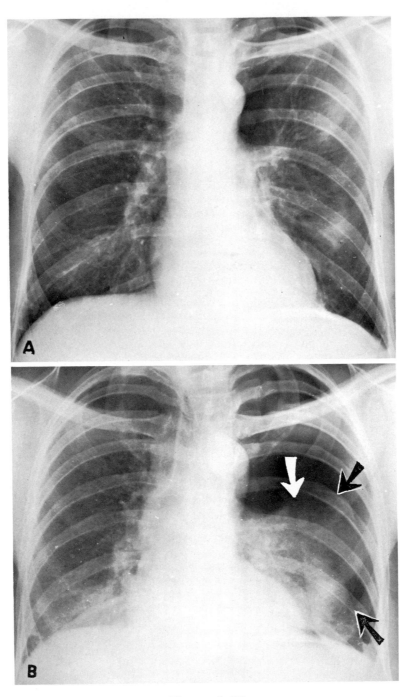

Figure l–11

26   **26**

A pneumothorax always appears larger on expiration than on inspiration. Since the thorax is (smaller
/ larger) on expiration, the unchanged volume of
pleural air spreads out in the smaller thoracic space.
Occasionally a small pneumothorax is *only* visible on
expiration.   smaller

Figure 1-11, *A*, is an inspiratory film. A definite pneumothorax is not
seen. Figure 1-11, *B*, is an expiratory film made immediately after *A*,
showing a large left pneumothorax (arrows outline the compressed
lung).

27   **27**

Let's go on to another concept. Three things happen
to the x-ray beam after it enters a patient:

A. Some rays are scattered or deflected.

B. Some are partly absorbed by the body organs
    and tissues, in varying amounts, before reach-
    ing the film.

C. Some pass directly to the film without being   B. The variability of tis-
    affected by the patient.   sue and organ absorp-
                                                          tion is what causes the
Which of these is responsible for creating the   different "shadows"
images on an x-ray film? _____   we see.

The scattered radiation (A) produces a hazy, unsharp image, or fog, and
detracts from film clarity. The rays that pass directly through the
patient (C) merely blacken the film.

28   **28**

The portion of the beam that strikes the patient and
then is haphazardly deflected is called _____
radiation. This type of radiation is greater in   scattered
(obese / thin) patients.   obese

29

It is advantageous to reduce the amount of this
_____ radiation since it gives us no useful
information and "fogs" the film.

29

scattered

30

A grid, which is a large thin plate, is composed of
evenly spaced parallel strips of lead. These strips of
lead permit most of the perpendicular x-rays to reach
the film but absorb many of the obliquely scattered
x-rays. Thus, most of the scattered radiation is
absorbed when a _____ is used.

30

grid

31

Of course, some of the perpendicular rays strike the
lead strips and are absorbed, causing lines (grid lines)
to appear on the film. These grid lines tend to
(enhance / detract from) film clarity.

31

detract from

32

When a time-exposure photograph of a street scene
is made, moving cars are not visible. By the same
principle, if the grid is made to move during the
x-ray exposure, the grid lines (will / will not) be
seen.   The roentgenogram made with the moving
_____ is called a *Bucky* film, named
for Gustav Bucky, one of the discoverers of this
principle.

32

will not

grid

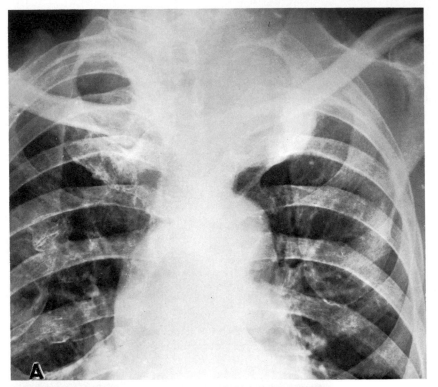

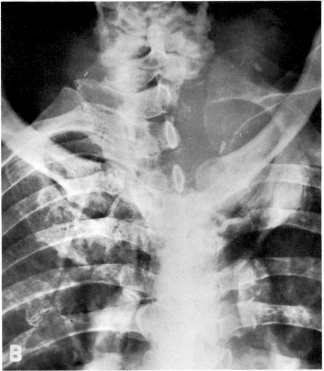

Figure 1–12

33

33

Thus, the purpose of a grid, fixed or moving, is to
absorb _____ radiation. The normal
lung, because of its gas content, gives off little of
this radiation, so a grid is not ordinarily required.
To better delineate a thick pulmonary or pleural   scattered
lesion, or the bony structures, however, it is often
helpful to obtain a _____ film.   Bucky

Figure 1-12, *A*, is a routine PA teleo showing a mass in the left apex.
Figure 1-12, *B*, a Bucky film, shows striking destruction of the upper
spine and ribs, indicating malignancy. Can you recognize it in ret-
rospect in *A*?

34

34

The moving grid, or _____ film, is   Bucky
usually utilized for detailed study of (thin / thick)
pulmonary or pleural lesions, or for depicting the   thick
_____ structures.
                                                       bony

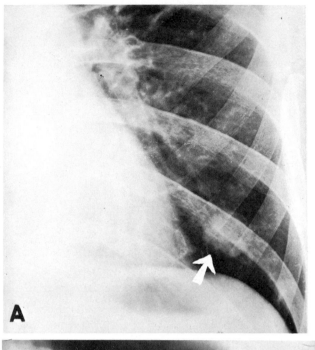

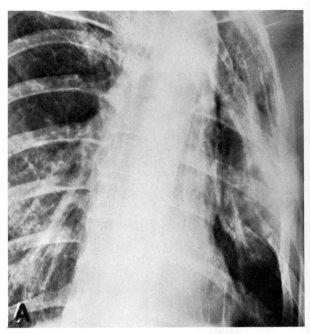

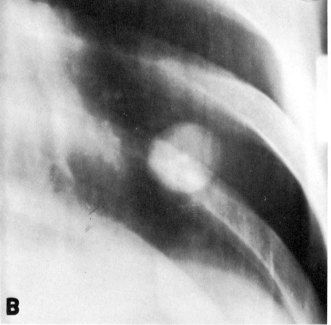

Figure 1-13

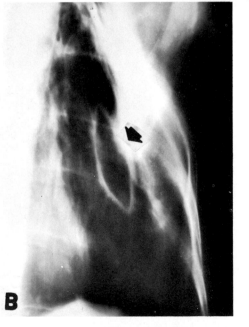

Figure 1-14

35

Another important technique is *laminagraphy*, also called *tomography*. With this method, radiographs of a desired layer of the body are obtained, at the same time blurring out structures in front of and behind this layer. This method, known as _____ , is especially helpful in evaluating pulmonary nodules, demonstrating cavities, and depicting bronchial obstruction.

laminagraphy
(tomography)

In Figure 1-13, the routine film (*A*) shows an apparently uncalcified nodule at the left lung base. In *B*, a laminagram, the nodule is seen better because the overlying ribs are blurred out. A central calcification is evident, indicating that it is a granuloma and not a tumor. Figure 1-14, *A*, shows a thoracoplasty (for tuberculosis), but no cavity is visible to explain the recurrence of a positive sputum. In *B*, the laminagram, the ribs are blurred out and a cavity is a clearly seen (arrow).

36

The principle of laminagraphy is simple. Let's perform another lamp experiment. Place a small light source directly over a piece of paper and hold your finger about 2 inches above the paper. Now, keeping your finger steady, move the light transversely at right angles to the finger. The shadow of the finger moves in the (same / opposite) direction as the light.

opposite

37

The light, finger, and shadow move as if connected by a rigid rod, with the finger as a fulcrum. If the paper could be moved in the same direction and at exactly the same speed as the shadow, the shadow would (always / seldom) fall on the same spot on the paper. So it would (always / seldom) be in focus.

always

always

38

Now, repeat the experiment but use two fingers, one about an inch above the other. As the light is moved, the shadows of the 2 fingers move (equally / unequally). If the paper could be moved synchronously with the shadow of one finger, the shadow of the other finger would be (in focus / blurred).

38

unequally

blurred

39

The laminagraph consists of an apparatus in which the tube and film move synchronously but in opposite directions. The adjustable fulcrum is set to the plane of the lesion to be studied. Structures in the planes above and below this level are _____ but the plane of the fulcrum remains in sharp focus. It's like taking x-ray slices through the patient!

39

blurred

REVIEW

I

Which view or technique, other than the routine PA and lateral, would give the most information in the following situations?

(a) Free pleural fluid on the right:
   **

(b) Questionable pneumonia in the lingula:
   **

(c) Tuberculosis at the left apex:
   **

(d) Bilateral encapsulated pleural fluid:
   **

I

(a) right lateral decubitus
   (See Figure 1-4.)

(b) lordotic
   (See Figure 1-8.)

(c) lordotic
   (See Figure 1-7.)

(d) both oblique views
   (See Figure 1-3.)

(e) Suspected obstructive emphysema:
**
_____

(f) Best visualization of the lateral wall of a left lung abscess:
**
_____

(e) expiration
(See Figure 1-10.)

(f) right lateral decubitus
(See Figure 1-5.)

II

List 2 indications for a Bucky film:
**
_____
**
_____

II

To better delineate:
(1) A thick pulmonary lesion
(2) A thick pleural lesion
(3) A bone lesion

III

List 2 indications for laminagraphy:
**
_____
**
_____

III

(1) Evaluation of a pulmonary nodule
(2) Demonstration of cavitation
(3) Demonstration of bronchial obstruction

Chapter 2 | LOBAR ANATOMY

1

As the years pass, anatomic details are quickly forgotten — even the Bardot variety. Nonetheless, a finger-tip knowledge of simple lobar and segmental anatomy is absolutely essential for chest roentgen interpretation.

We challenge you to test your anatomic recall:

(a) Which lung is the larger?

_____

(b) Name the lobes of the left lung.

_____

(c) Name the lobes of the right lung.

_____

1

(a) the right. The heart encroaches more on the left lung.

(b) upper, lower

(c) upper, middle, lower

2

Each lobe is covered by *visceral* pleura. The visceral pleura bordering adjacent surfaces of two lobes form the *septa*, which separate the _____ .

2

lobes

> The space between 2 adjacent septa is called an *interlobar fissure*. Get the distinction? A fissure is a narrow space; a septum is a divider. Examples: nasal septum, anal fissure. If in doubt, palpate.
> The 2 terms, fissure and septum, are actually used interchangeably in the thorax, and we will do so from now on.

3

Adjacent lobes are separated by an interlobar _____ .

3

septum or fissure (Remember, we use the terms interchangeably.)

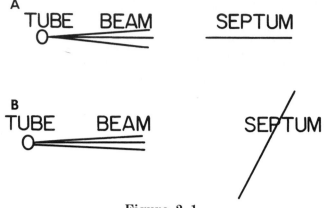

Figure 2–1

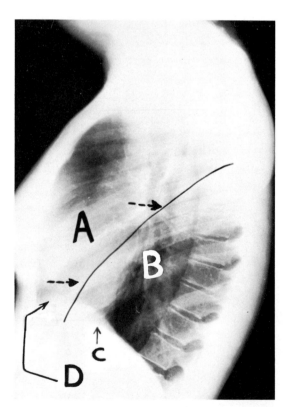

Figure 2–2. On this and many subsequent illustrations, we have indicated the position of the interlobar fissures by black lines because these structures are difficult to reproduce.

4

4

Since a septum is less than 1 mm. thick, the x-ray beam must strike it parallel to the long axis if it is to be visible on the roentgenogram. If a septum is not _____ to the x-ray beam, it will not be visualized.

parallel

This frame embodies a concept that is used in all phases of roentgenology. So we recommend that you read it again.

5

5

In Figure 2-1, *A*, the x-ray beam is _____ to the septum. There (will / will not) be a shadow of the septum on the roentgenogram.

parallel

will

In Figure 2-1, *B*, the x-ray beam (is / is not) parallel to the septum. There (will / will not) be a shadow of the septum on the roentgenogram.

is not

will not

6

6

The oblique or major fissure of the left lung separates the upper lobe from the _____ _____ .

lower lobe

7

7

Figure 2-2 shows that in the left lung the upper lobe, A, is separated from the lower lobe, B, by the _____ _____ (broken arrows). C denotes the diaphragm, and D the anterior costophrenic angle.

major (oblique) fissure

8

8

Figure 2-2 shows that the _____ fissure runs obliquely downward from about the level of the fifth thoracic vertebra to the _____ at a point just behind the anterior costophrenic angle.

major (oblique)

diaphragm

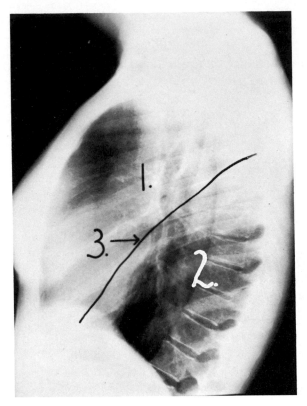

Figure 2-3

9

9

The oblique fissure is ordinarily not visible on the normal frontal projection because (*choose one*):

(a) It is often anatomically absent.
(b) It is not parallel to the x-ray beam.
(c) It has the same roentgen density as lung tissue.

(b) It is not parallel to the x-ray beam.

10

10

On the left lateral view (Figure 2-3), indentify the following lobes:

(1) _____
(2) _____

(1) upper

(2) lower

What is the arrow (3) pointing to ?
(3) _____ _____

(3) major fissure

11

11

In the right lung, the major fissure separates the upper and middle lobes from the _____
_____.

lower lobe

Except for this, what has been said about the left major fissure applies also to the right.

12

12

In the lateral view, the intersection of the major fissure with its hemidiaphragm is often seen. By identifying which hemidiaphragm is which (from the gastric air bubble, bottom of the heart, and other signs), one can identify the corresponding major fissure. This isn't very important, so forget it. (Bet you can't now.)

By the way, this frame is on us.

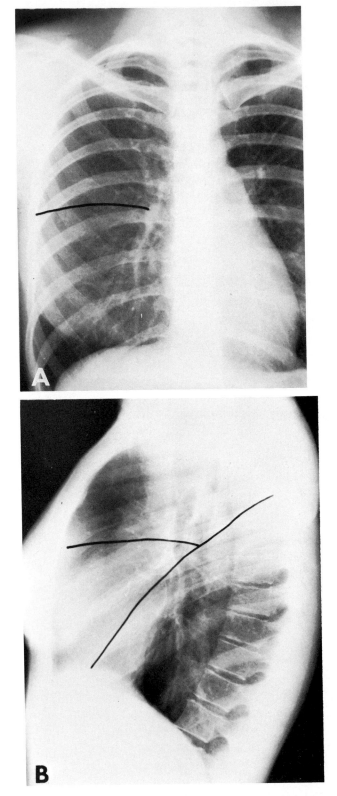

Figure 2–4

13   **13**

Now, let's go on to another important fissure. The
minor or horizontal fissure separates the middle lobe
from the (left / right) upper lobe.   right

We apologize for insulting your intelligence.

14   **14**

Since the minor fissure is parallel to the floor (Figure
2-4, *A* & *B*), and so is the x-ray beam, this fissure
(will / will not) be visible in *both* frontal and lateral
views.   will

15   **15**

Figure 2-4, *B*, shows that the minor fissure runs   anterior
from the _____ chest wall to intersect
the _____ _____.   major fissure

16   **16**

The position of the minor fissure is variable. The
lower the position of the minor fissure, the (larger
/ smaller) is the middle lobe.   smaller

The minor fissure may intersect the lateral chest wall anywhere between
the anterior portion of the second and sixth ribs, but most often
intersects it at about the level of the fourth rib.

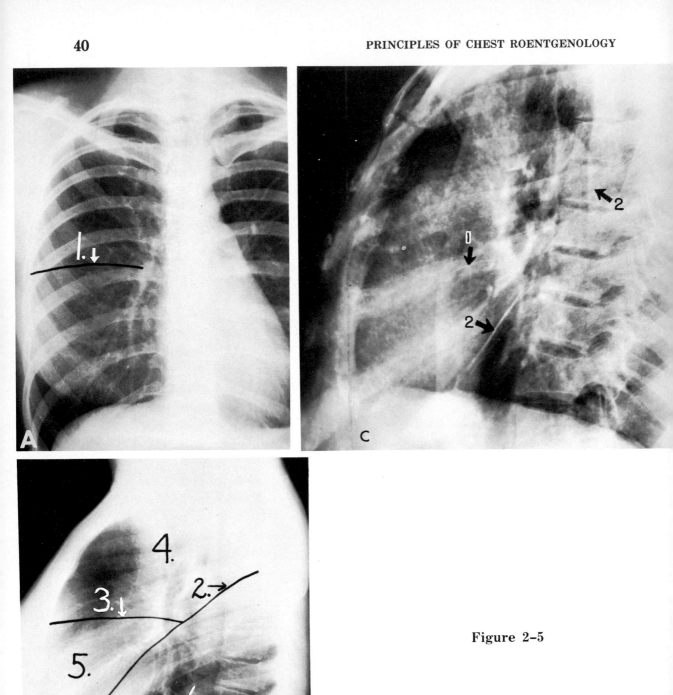

Figure 2-5

17   17

More exceptions:

The minor fissure is anatomically absent or incomplete in 25 per cent of individuals.

Also, if it happens to be tilted, the x-ray beam may not be _____ to it, and the fissure will not be seen.

parallel

The minor fissure was not visible at all in the PA roentgenograms of 44 per cent of 1000 healthy adults. The same figure should hold for unhealthy adults.

---

18   18

Identify the following on Figure 2-5, A & B:

(1) _____ _____   (1) minor fissure

(2) _____ _____   (2) major fissure

(3) _____ _____   (3) minor fissure

(4) ** _____   (4) right upper lobe

(5) ** _____   (5) right middle lobe

(6) ** _____   (6) right lower lobe

Figure 2-5, C, is an unretouched illustration of the right fissures.

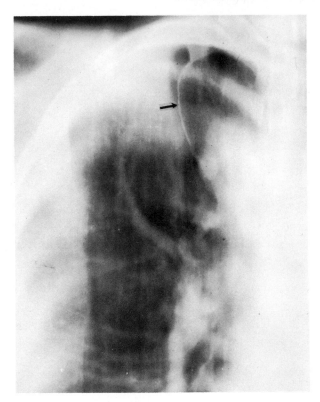

Figure 2-6

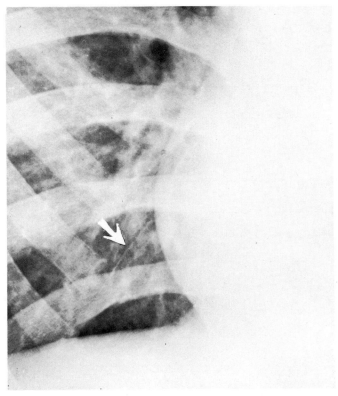

Figure 2-7

19

Now, what about other fissures? The azygos lobe
(Figure 2-6), is formed by an anomalous development
of the azygos vein, which "cuts through" the right
upper lobe. The azygos lobe is separated from the
rest of the upper lobe by the azygos _____
(arrow).

19

fissure

It is practically never seen in the left lung for the simple reason that
normally there ain't no azygos vein on the left.

20

The azygos fissure subtends a variable amount of
the upper medial region of the _____
_____ lobe. This portion of the lung is called
the _____ lobe.

20

right upper

azygos

It is visible in about 1 of 200 normal individuals. Watch for it.

21

Figure 2-7 shows the position of another anomalous
fissure (arrow), seen in about 5 per cent of normal
individuals. It is the inferior accessory fissure,
which separates the medial basal segment of the
_____ lobe from the remainder of the
lobe.

21

lower

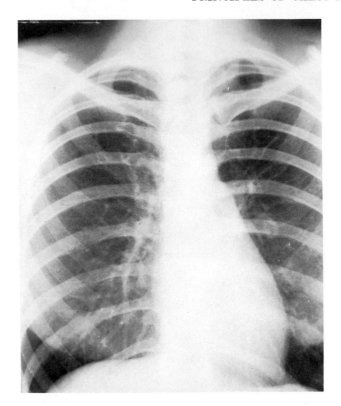

Figure 2-8

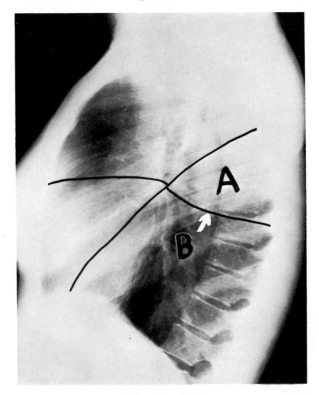

Figure 2-9

22

The fissure that separates the medial basal segment of the lower lobe from the remainder of the lobe is called the _____ _____ fissure. Draw its location on Figure 2-8. While you're at it, draw the minor fissure too.

22

inferior accessory

Compare your lines with those in Figure 2-7 and in Figure 2-4, *A*.

23

Now imagine the x-ray beam striking the inferior accessory fissure from the lateral direction. Should you see it in the lateral view?
   (Obviously yes! / Definitely not!)

23

Definitely not!

If you answered Frame 23 incorrectly you had better turn back to Frame 4 and re-read the basic concept.

24

The minor, azygos, and inferior accessory fissures are often seen in the _____ lung but hardly ever in the _____ lung.

24

right

left

25

The superior accessory fissure separates the superior segment of either lower lobe from the remainder of the lower lobe in about 5 per cent of anatomic specimens. In Figure 2-9, A represents the superior segment of the right lower lobe. What is B ?
   ** _____

25

superior accessory fissure

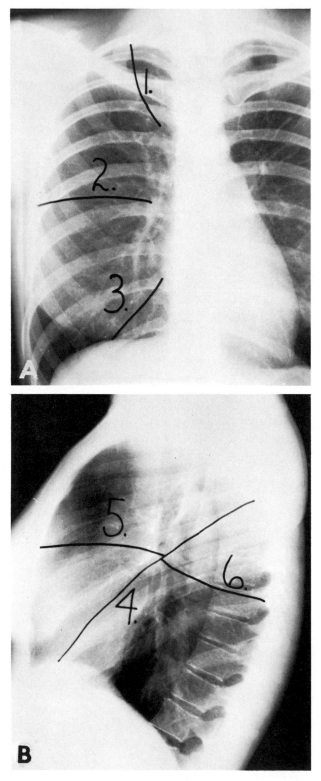

Figure 2–10

26   26

The _____ accessory fissure may be
visible on both the frontal and lateral views, because   superior
it is _____ to the floor. On the
frontal view, it is usually mistaken for the   parallel
_____ fissure, since both these fissures lie at
about the same level.   minor

> However, in the lateral view the minor fissure is anterior and the
> superior accessory fissure is posterior. If you had trouble with Frame
> 26, refer back to Figure 2-9.

REVIEW

Identify the fissures in Figure 2-10, *A & B*:   (1) azygos

   (1) _____   (2) minor or superior
   (2) _____ or _____ _____   accessory
   (3) _____ _____
   (4) _____   (3) inferior accessory
   (5) _____
   (6) _____ _____   (4) major

                                                              (5) minor

                                                              (6) superior accessory

> Train yourself to look for the fissures on *every* roentgenogram of the
> chest. As we shall see, displacement of the fissures is the most reliable
> sign of lobar collapse.

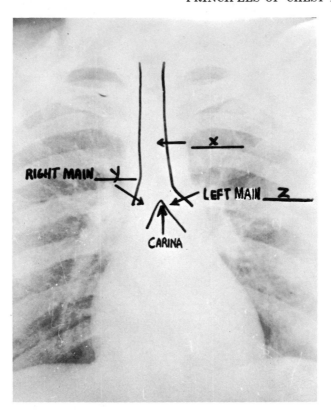

Figure 3-1

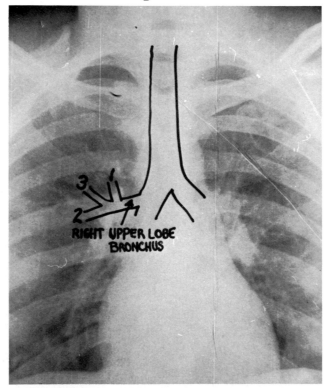

Figure 3-2

Chapter 3

SEGMENTAL ANATOMY

A knowledge of the segmental anatomy of the lung is indispensable for identifying bronchial orifices and extracting foreign bodies at bronchoscopy, for finding lesions at the operating table, for prescribing appropriate postural drainage of pulmonary abscess, and for differential diagnosis. Some conditions have a segmental distribution; others do not. Some diseases are commonly found in a particular segment; others almost never. So you can see why we think segmental anatomy is essential to an understanding of chest roentgenology.

1

Each lobe of the lung is divided into segments, which can readily be stripped apart. Each segment is supplied by its own bronchus, which is called a segmental bronchus.

1

For free.

2

The structures drawn in Figure 3-1 should be familiar to you. Fill in the blanks:

(x) _____
(y) _____
(z) _____

2

(x) trachea

(y) bronchus

(z) bronchus

3

Let's start with the right upper lobe (RUL). In Figure 3-2 the RUL bronchus is shown. Note that this bronchus comes off at about the level of the tracheal bifurcation (carina). The RUL bronchus normally has 3 segmental branches which lead to the 3 _____ of the RUL.

3

segments

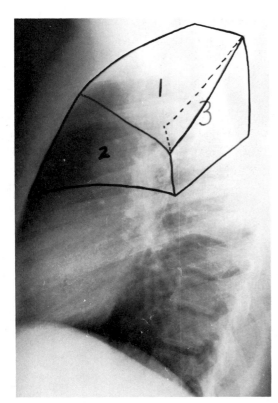

Figure 3–3

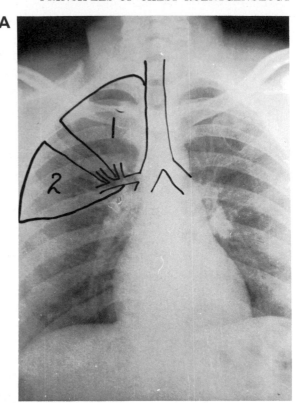

A

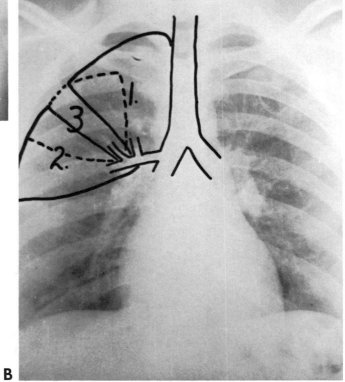

B

Figure 3–4

4

Figure 3-3, a lateral diagram, shows the 3 segments of the RUL, each numbered. These numbers follow the bronchial numbering system of Boyden (an anatomist now living in Seattle). The actual numbers are important, both in this program and in the literature. These numbers are always assigned in the order of the take-off of the segmental bronchi from the lobar bronchus. In Figure 3-3, #1 is the *apical* segment, #2 is the *anterior* segment, and, obviously, #3 is the _____ segment.

4

posterior

(Where does that anatomist live? _____)

5

Here are Boyden's numbers for the segments of the RUL. Name each of them:

#1. _____
#2. _____
#3. _____

We will use Boyden's numbering system exclusively. (Don't forget his address.)

5

#1. apical

#2. anterior

#3. posterior

6

Figure 3-4, *A & B*, shows the location of these segments on the PA view. Note the overlap of the segments — that's the trouble with the PA view for studying segmental anatomy. Number the segments according to _____ system:

_____ posterior
_____ apical
_____ anterior

6

Boyden's

#3

#1

#2

The anterior segment of an upper lobe is only rarely the site of a solitary focus of tuberculosis, whereas carcinoma of the lung is frequently found there.

A

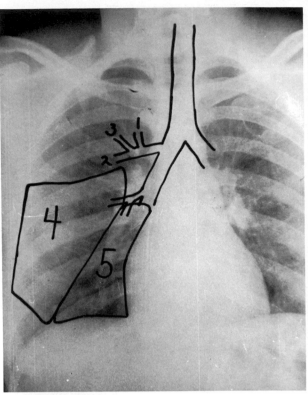

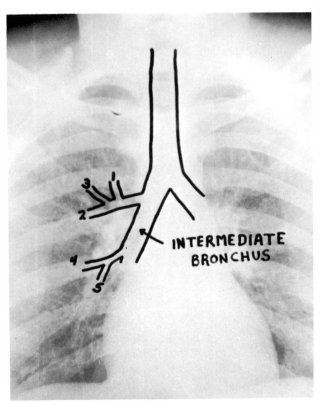

Figure 3–5

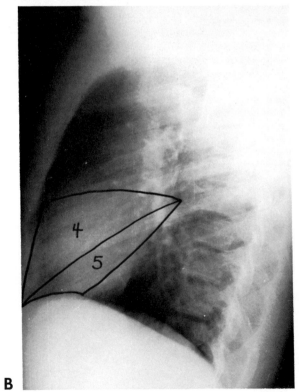

B

Figure 3–6

7

Look at Figure 3-5. The intermediate bronchus is
the continuation of the right _____
bronchus after the _____ bronchus
takes off.

7

main

RUL

8

The right middle lobe (RML) bronchus arises from
the intermediate bronchus and divides into 2 segmental bronchi: #4, the lateral segment, and #5, the
medial segment. Name all of the numbered segments
on Figure 3-5:

    #1. _____
    #2. _____
    #3. _____
    #4. _____
    #5. _____

    It's not so tough, is it?

8

#1. apical ⎫
#2. anteror ⎬ RUL
#3. posterior ⎭

#4. lateral ⎫ RML
#5. medial ⎭

9

PA and lateral views of the RML are diagrammed
and numbered on Figure 3-6, *A & B*. Indicate the
names of:

    #4. _____
    #5. _____

9

#4. lateral

#5. medial

10

The right lower lobe (RLL) bronchus is the continuation of the intermediate bronchus below the take-off
of the _____ bronchus.

10

RML

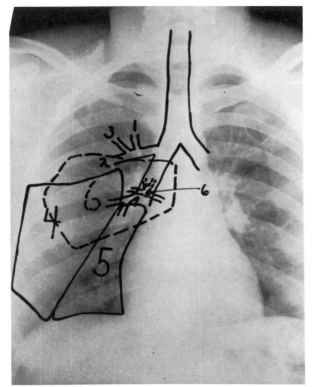

Figure 3-7

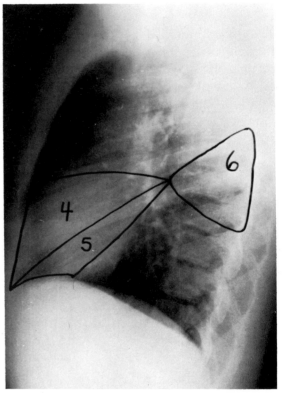

Figure 3-8

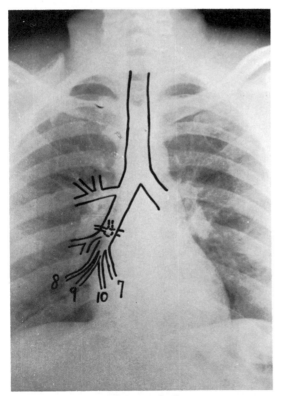

Figure 3-9

11

The highest segmental bronchus of the RLL arises posteriorly, just opposite the RML bronchus. It is labeled #6 in Figure 3-7, and supplies the superior segment of the right _____ lobe.

11

lower

12

Figures 3-7 and 3-8 show the anatomic position of segment #6, which is the _____ segment of the RLL.

12

superior

Lung abscess is common in this segment.

13

The 4 remaining segmental bronchi supply the 4 *basal* segments of the RLL. They are numbered in the order of their origin from the parent bronchus (see Figure 3-9). They are very logically named. Segment #7 is the medial basal segment and #8 is the anterior basal segment. Guess what #9 and #10 are called. (Remember, be logical.)

  # 9. _____ _____
  #10. _____ _____

13

9. lateral basal

#10. posterior basal

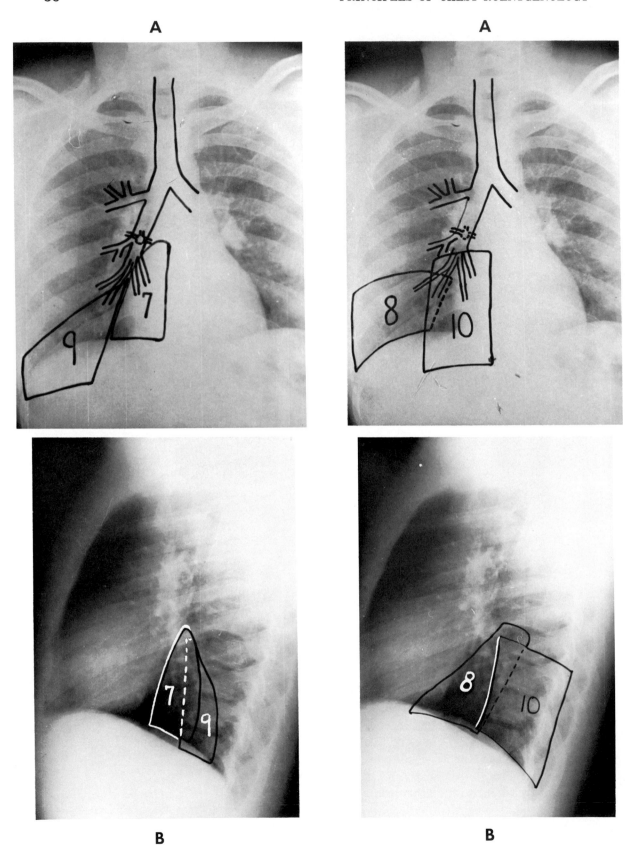

A

A

B

B

Figure 3–10

Figure 3–11

14   **14**

Figure 3-10, *A & B*, show the position of segments
#7 and #9.

                                  #7. medial basal

    #7 is the _____ _____

    #9 is the _____ _____   #9. lateral basal

Note that they overlap in the lateral view.

15   **15**

Figure 3-11, *A & B*, shows the position of segments
#8 and #10.

                                  # 8. anterior basal

    # 8 is the _____ _____

    #10 is the _____ _____   #10. posterior basal

    By the way, what is #6 again? _____   # 6. superior

Note in Figure 3-11, *A*, that the anterior and posterior basal segments
overlap in the PA view, but the posterior segment is a bit lower.

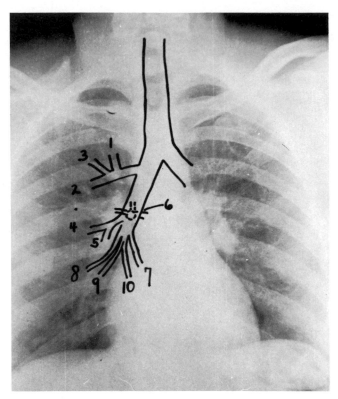

Figure 3–12

16

Name all the segmental bronchi of the right lung indicated in Figure 3-12:

1. _____
2. _____
3. _____
4. _____
5. _____
6. _____
7. _____ _____
8. _____ _____
9. _____ _____
#10. _____ _____

16

1. apical
2. anterior   } RUL
3. posterior

4. lateral   } RML
5. medial

6. superior
7. medial basal
8. anterior
        basal   } RLL
9. lateral basal
#10. posterior
        basal

17

Name all the segments in the right lung without their Boyden numbers:

_____
_____
_____
_____
_____
_____
_____ _____
_____ _____
_____ _____
_____ _____

17

RUL { apical
      anterior
      posterior

RML { lateral
      medial

RLL { superior
      medial basal
      anterior basal
      lateral basal
      posterior basal

18

Here's a segmental scramble. Fill in the blanks:

#9. _____ _____
_____ anterior
_____ medial
#6. _____
_____ medial basal
#4. _____

18

#9. lateral basal
#2. anterior
#5. medial
#6. superior
#7. medial basal
#4. lateral

A

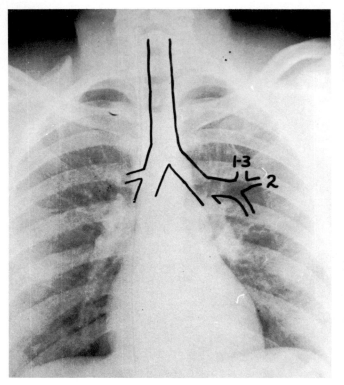

Figure 3–13

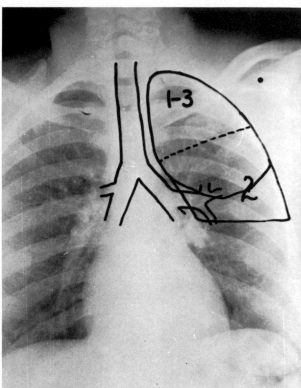

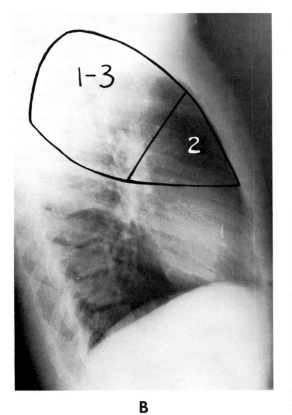

B

Figure 3–14

19

Have you noted in the illustrations how much the segments overlap each other in the frontal view? The left oblique and _____ views are better for recognizing the segments, since there is little overlap in these projections.

lateral

The right oblique and lateral views are best for the left lung for the same reason.

20

O.K., you are now ready to learn the segmental anatomy of the left lung. The differences between the 2 lungs are minor, so don't get discouraged. Remember that no paired organs are symmetrical — not even the testes.

First of all there are only 2 lobes on the left, the _____ lobe and the _____ lobe. The homologue of the RML is called the *lingula*.

upper

lower

21

As on the right side, the first bronchus arising from the left main bronchus is the left _____ _____ bronchus. It divides into an upper and lower (lingular) division (Figure 3-13).

upper lobe

22

The upper division of the LUL has only 2 segments: #1-3, the apical posterior — which is the counterpart of the apical (#1) and posterior (#3) segments of the RUL—and #2, the _____ segment.

Figure 3-14, *A & B*, shows these segments in PA and lateral projection. The dotted line in *A* represents the top of segment #2.

anterior

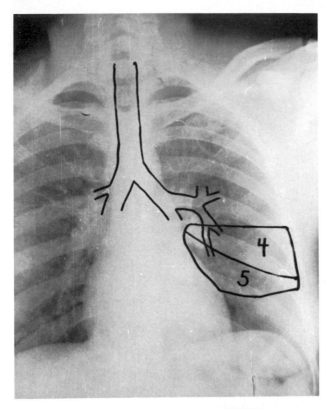

Figure 3–15

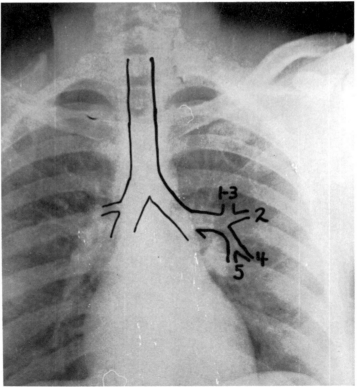

Figure 3–16

23

The lower or lingular division of the LUL is subdivided into 2 segments: #4, the superior lingular and #5, the _____ lingular. These segments are shown in Figure 3-15. Note that the lingula is similar in position to the right _____ lobe. While you're at it, name and number the 2 segments of the RML:

_____ _____
_____ _____

23

inferior

middle

#4. lateral ⎫
                    ⎬ RML
#5. medial ⎭

24

List the names of all the segments of the LUL indicated in Figure 3-16:

#1-3. _____ _____
#2. _____
#4. _____ _____
#5. _____ _____

24

#1-3. apical posterior

#2. anterior

#4. superior lingular

#5. inferior lingular

25

The RML bronchus arises from the _____ bronchus. The lingular bronchus arises from the _____ bronchus.

25

intermediate

LUL

Useless information: There is no intermediate bronchus in the left lung. You're welcome.

26   26

Guess what — the LLL has the same segmental anatomy as the right! (Some authorities don't agree with this statement, but they're wrong and we and Boyden are right.) Using your power of total recall, number and name the segments of the LLL and tell us the capital of the state of Washington:

6. superior

7. medial basal

8. anterior basal

9. lateral basal

#10. posterior basal

_____ _____
_____ _____ _____
_____ _____ _____
_____ _____ _____
_____ _____ _____
The capital of Washington is _____ .

Olympia, you dummkopf!

REVIEW

The segmental anatomy, as we have presented it, is "idealized." There is considerable variation from patient to patient in the size and distribution of the segments. But the basic patterns are generally present. Name and number all the segments of each lung:

Right lung   Right lung

_____ _____   # 1. apical
_____ _____   # 2. anterior
_____ _____   # 3. posterior
_____ _____   # 4. lateral
_____ _____   # 5. medial
_____ _____   # 6. superior
_____ _____ _____   # 7. medial basal
_____ _____ _____   # 8. anterior basal
_____ _____ _____   # 9. lateral basal
_____ _____ _____   #10. posterior basal

Left lung	Left lung

Left lung

_____ _____ _____
_____ _____
_____ _____ _____
_____ _____ _____
_____ _____
_____ _____ _____
_____ _____ _____
_____ _____ _____
_____ _____ _____

Left lung

#1-3. apical posterior
2. anterior
4. superior lingular
5. inferior lingular
6. superior
7. medial basal
8. anterior basal
9. lateral basal
#10. posterior basal

Well, you've got it now — but how long will you remember it? This depends on how often you use it. From now on try to localize all lung lesions you see in terms of segments. Check your localizations with a radiologist.

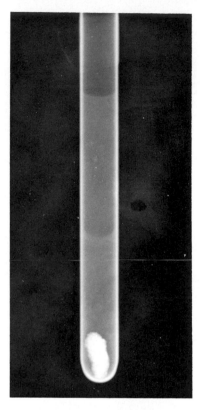

Figure 4-1

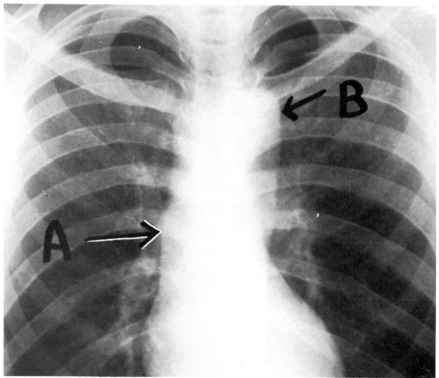

Figure 4-2

THE SILHOUETTE SIGN

Chapter 4

1

1

There are 4 basic roentgen densities: gas, water, fat, and metal. In order of *increasing* density they are gas, fat, water, and _____.

metal

Figure 4-1 shows a test tube containing, from top down, air, oil (fat), water, and metal. Calcium is the prime example of metal density *normally* found in the body.

2

2

Anatomic structures are recognized on the roentgenogram by their differences in density. The 4 basic densities keep the radiologist in business. A normal chest film, Figure 4-2, shows them as the water density of the heart, muscles, and blood; the metal (calcium) density of the ribs; the _____ density of the lungs; and streaks of fat density around the muscles (not shown).

gas (air)

In Figure 4-2 the ascending aorta and aortic knob (posterior portion of aortic arch) are labeled: A — ascending aorta; B — aortic knob. Both are water density.

3

3

The heart, which is _____ density, can be differentiated from the ribs because the ribs are _____ density.

water

metal

67

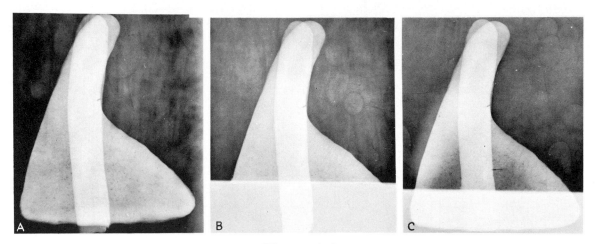

Figure 4-3

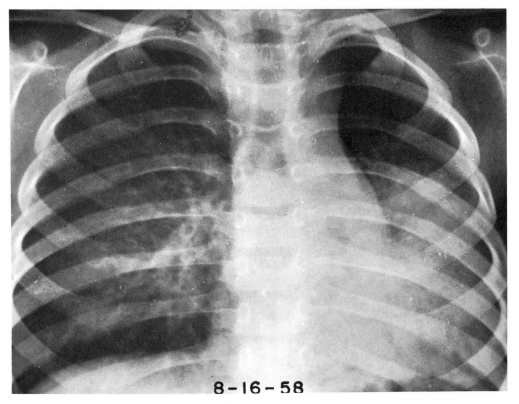

Figure 4-4

4

The heart, aorta, and blood, as well as the liver, spleen, and muscles, are all water density. So is diseased *airless* lung. Two substances of water density, when side by side, cannot be differentiated from each other. It is for this reason that the blood in the heart cannot be visualized, since both blood and heart are _____ density. So we have to inject a contrast medium (a metallic solution) to see the interior of the heart.

4

water

5

The 4 basic roentgen densities are:

_____

_____

_____

_____

5

air

fat

water

metal

6

Figure 4-3, *A*, is a roentgenogram of a model of the heart and aorta.* The heart and ascending aorta have been placed in one box and the aortic knob (posterior arch) and descending aorta in a second box, behind the first. In *B*, some water has been poured into the anterior box. The lower part of the heart has disappeared, but the descending aorta is still visible. In *C*, the water has been removed to the posterior box. What has happened to the lower descending aorta? ** _____

Is the entire heart visible? _____

6

It has disappeared.

Yes

7

Thus, a water density in *anatomic* contact with another water density obliterates the existing interface. Pneumonia (water density) in anatomic contact with a heart border (_____ density) will _____ that border.

7

water

obliterate

Figure 4-4 shows the left heart border obliterated by lingular pneumonia.

*Courtesy Dr. E. Martinez, Prescott, Arizona.

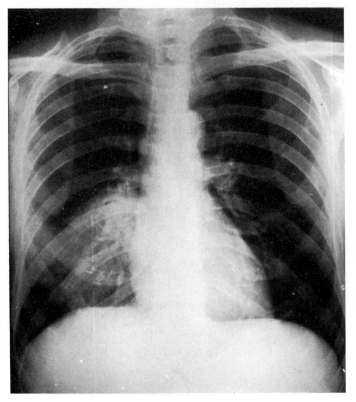

Figure 4–5

8

Similarly, a lesion of water density in anatomic contact with the aorta or diaphragm will _____ the border along the zone of contact. This phenomenon, the *loss* of the normal roentgen silhouette, is known as the **silhouette sign**.

8

obliterate

9

The silhouette sign is seen when a border of the heart, aorta, or _____ is obliterated.

9

diaphragm

10

Water density that is *not* in contact with the heart, the _____, or the diaphragm will *not* obliterate the border; and the silhouette sign is (absent / present).

10

aorta

absent

Figure 4-5 shows infiltrate that is not in anatomic contact with the right heart border, even though in this view it seems to be. Note that the right heart border is *not* obliterated by this RLL pneumonia.

11

Now that you know what the silhouette sign is, what are you going to do with it? O.K., we'll show you. Since the heart is an anterior structure in the chest, obviously both its right and left borders are also _____ in location. So is the ascending aorta.

11

anterior

12

The right heart border, left heart border, and ascending aorta, then, are all _____ structures.

12

anterior

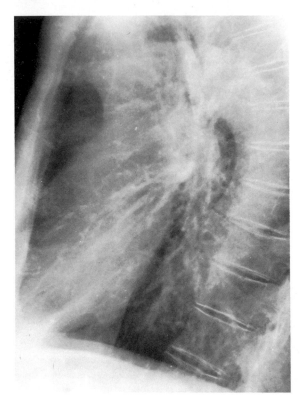

Figure 4-6

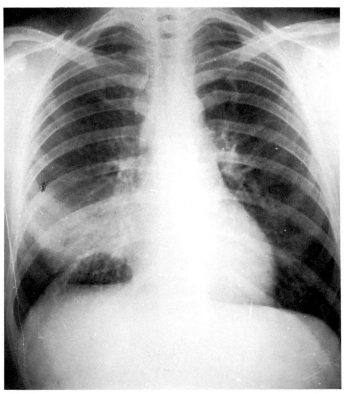

Figure 4-7

13   **13**

The aortic knob (posterior part of the aortic arch)
and the descending thoracic aorta are posterior
structures.   The ascending aorta is _____   anterior
but the descending aorta and aortic knob are
_____ in location.   posterior

Figure 4-6 is a lateral view of the chest, which shows the anterior position of the heart and ascending aorta and the posterior position of the
aortic knob and descending aorta.

14   **14**

Let's wrap this up.   State the anterior or posterior   (a) posterior
location of each of the following:
                                                              (b) anterior

  (a) aortic knob   _____   (c) posterior
  (b) right heart border _____
  (c) descending aorta   _____   (d) anterior
  (d) left heart border _____
  (e) ascending aorta   _____   (e) anterior

15   **15**

Now, the RML lies in anatomic contact with all but
the uppermost portion of the right heart border.
Since the right heart border is an anterior structure, the RML must be an _____
structure (which we knew anyhow).   anterior

16   **16**

The lobe of the lung in contact with the greater
part of the right heart border is the _____.   RML

17   **17**

If the right heart border is obliterated by a lung
lesion, the silhouette sign tells us that the lesion is   anterior
_____ and is located in the
_____.   See what we're driving at?   RML

Figure 4-7 shows obliteration of the right heart border by pneumonia
in the RML.   Compare with Figure 4-5.

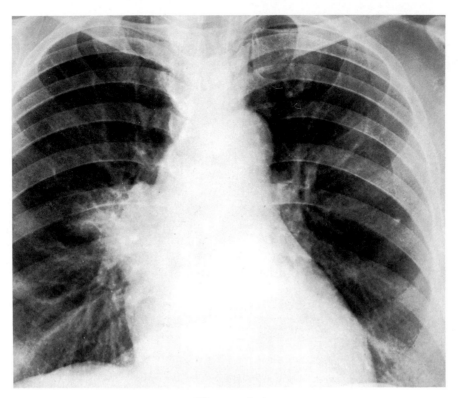

Figure 4-8

18

The uppermost portion of the right heart border and the ascending aorta are in anatomic contact with the anterior segment of the RUL (Boyden #2). Since the right heart border and ascending aorta are _____, the anterior segment of the right upper lobe must also be anterior. Sound silly? You'll see.

18

anterior

Figure 4-8 shows obliteration of the upper right heart border and ascending aorta by pneumonia in the anterior segment of the RUL.

19

The ascending aorta and *upper* portion of the right heart border are in contact with the _____ _____ of the RUL.

19

anterior segment (#2)

20

Disease in the anterior segment of the RUL may obliterate either the _____ _____ or
** _____ or both.

20

ascending aorta

right heart border (Remember, uppermost portion only.)

21

The lingula, which is really the left counterpart of the _____, lies in anatomic contact with the left heart border. Since the left heart border is _____ in location, the lingula is also _____.

21

RML

anterior

anterior

22

The portion of the lung in contact with the left heart border is the _____, and disease here will obliterate this border.

22

lingula

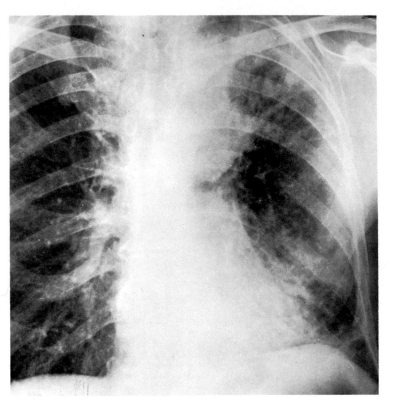

Figure 4–9

23

Now, let's summarize:
The lingula is in contact with the ** _____.
The right middle lobe is in contact with the
** _____. The anterior segment of the
right upper lobe is in contact with the _____
_____ and the uppermost portion of the
** _____.
Don't get annoyed. Repetition clinches facts
(cliché).

23

left heart border

right heart border

ascending aorta

right heart border

(It's easy, isn't it?)

24

The anterior segment of the LUL (#2) lies in contact with the upper portion of the left heart border.
The greater portion of the left heart border, however, is in contact with the _____.

24

lingula

Figure 4-9 shows obliteration of the left heart border by pneumonia
in the lingula. Ignore the upper half of the figure. (Bet you won't.)

25

If the following structures are obliterated, what lung
segment or lobe is involved?

(a) most of the left heart border

_____

(b) most of the right heart border

_____

(c) upper part of left heart border

_____

(d) ascending aorta

_____

(e) upper part of right heart border

_____

25

(a) lingula

(b) RML

(c) anterior segment,
    LUL (#2)

(d) anterior segment,
    RUL (#2)

(e) anterior segment,
    RUL (#2)

Rest for a couple of minutes if you want. (Bathroom? Just a reminder.)

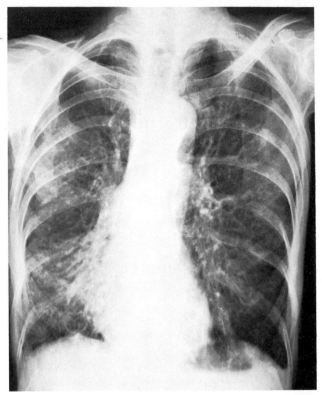

Figure 4–10

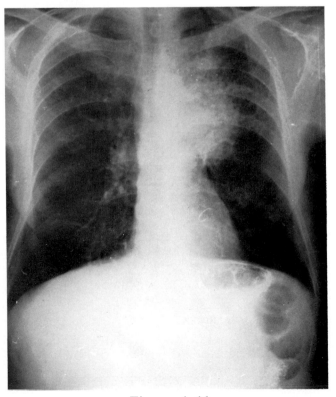

Figure 4–11

26

In Figure 4-10:

(a) Which heart border is obliterated? _____
(b) Is the disease anterior or posterior? _____
(c) What lobe is involved? _____

26

(a) right

(b) anterior

(c) RML

This patient has bronchiectasis of the RML with collapse.

27

The apical posterior segment of the LUL (#1-3) lies in anatomic contact with the aortic knob. The apical posterior segment and aortic knob are both _____ structures.

27

posterior

28

The apical posterior segment of the LUL (#1-3) lies in anatomic contact with the _____ _____.

28

aortic knob

Figure 4-11 shows obliteration of the aortic knob by a carcinoma in the apical posterior segment of the LUL. The upper portion of Figure 4-9 shows pneumonia in this same segment.

29

Pneumonia, tumor, or any other lesion of water density that obliterates the aortic knob is in the _____ _____ segment of the LUL. The aortic knob and this segment are alike in being _____ structures.

29

apical posterior (#1-3)

posterior

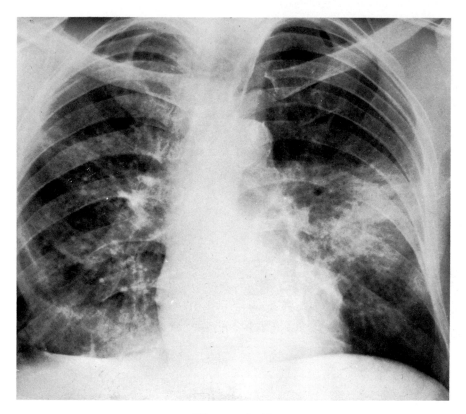

Figure 4–12

30

In Figure 4-12:

(a) What structure is obliterated?

_____

(b) Is the disease anterior or posterior?

_____

(c) In what anatomic location is this lesion?

_____

30

(a) left heart border

(b) anterior

(c) lingula (#4 and #5)

31

Now let's go after the lower lobes. The RLL and LLL are posterior structures. They are not in anatomic contact with the heart borders, which are _____ structures.

31

anterior

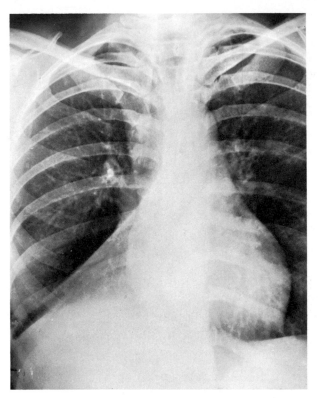

Figure 4–13

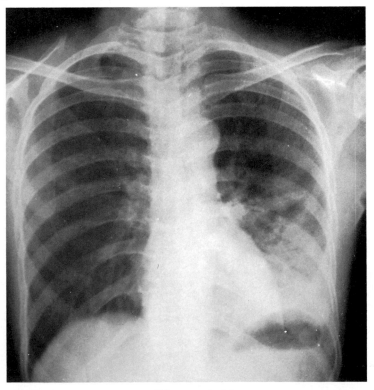

Figure 4–14

32

Disease in the RLL does *not* obliterate the _____

_____ _____.

Obviously the same principle holds true on the left
side.

32

right heart border

Figure 4-13 shows collapse of the RLL by carcinoma; the right heart
border is not obliterated.
    Figure 4-14 shows pneumonia in the LLL, which fails to obliterate
the left heart border.

33

If disease in the left lower lung obliterates the left
heart border, it lies in the _____; if
it overlaps but doesn't obliterate the heart border,
it lies in the _____.

33

lingula

LLL

34

Disease in the superior segment (#6) of either the
RLL or LLL will overlap the middle portion of the
heart border, but will not obliterate these borders
because the superior segments are _____
structures.

34

posterior

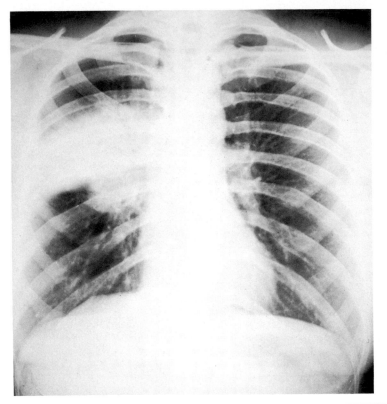

Figure 4–15

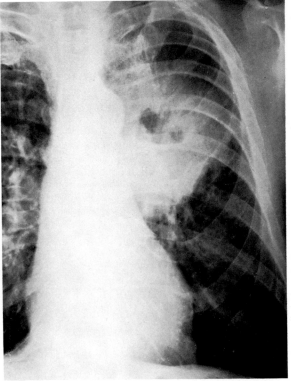

Figure 4–16

35   **35**

A lesion that overlaps but does not obliterate the
ascending aorta is _____ in location.   posterior

> Figure 4-15 shows an intact border of the ascending aorta overlapped
> by pneumonia in the superior segment (#6) of the RLL. We can see
> the ascending aorta. Can you?

36   **36**

The aortic knob and descending thoracic aorta are
_____ structures.   posterior

37   **37**

To obliterate the aortic knob or any part of the   descending
_____ thoracic aorta, the disease proc-
ess must be located _____.   posteriorly

38   **38**

Conversely, if the disease overlaps but does not
obliterate the aortic knob, it is located _____
to these structures.   anterior

> Hold it! It could also lie far posterior, *behind* the aortic knob, which
> isn't a very thick structure. Figure 4-16 shows an intact aortic knob
> in a patient with tuberculosis in the superior segment of the LLL.

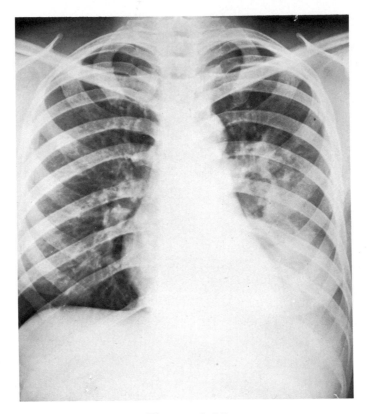

Figure 4–17

39

Now let's move to the diaphragm. Like the heart,
the diaphragm is of _____ density.
Disease of water density in anatomic contact with   water
the diaphragm will _____ its border.
This may be seen in either the PA or lateral view.   obliterate

39

Figure 4-17 shows obliteration of the left hemidiaphragm by LLL
tuberculosis. Note the visible left heart border.

40

In the lateral view the entire right hemidiaphragm
and the posterior half of the left hemidiaphragm are
visible. Obviously, the anterior part of the left
hemidiaphragm is _____, because   obliterated
there is anatomic contact between the _____
and the bottom of the heart.   hemidiaphragm

41

The anterior portion of which hemidiaphragm is
normally obliterated by the bottom of the heart?
_____   the left

42

You've learned that the silhouette sign applies to
lung lesions. It also applies to mediastinal lesions
and pleural fluid. For instance, an anterior mediastinal tumor in contact with the right heart border
will _____ that border.   obliterate

43

Pleural fluid encapsulated in the anterior pleural
cavity in _____ contact with a border
of the heart or ascending aorta will obliterate that
border.   anatomic

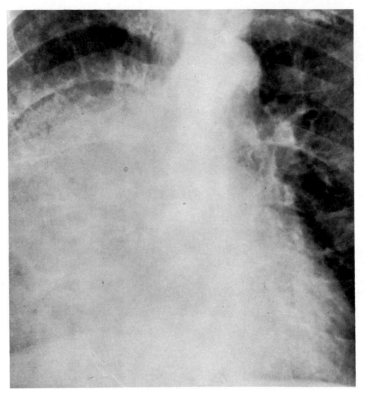

Figure 4–18

44

If the aortic knob or descending thoracic aorta is obliterated, the lesion causing this could lie in the lung, in the posterior pleural cavity, or in the _____ mediastinum.

44

posterior

45

Now everything is clear — but here come the exceptions. The silhouette sign may be misleading on an underpenetrated roentgenogram (a film that is too light). For instance, right lower lobe disease may appear to obliterate the right heart border on an underpenetrated film.

45

(Sorry, we forgot to leave a blank.)

46

Another exception: Sometimes the right heart border overlies the spine and doesn't protrude into the right lung field. The _____ density of the spine hides the area adjacent to the right heart border. You can't hit 'em if you can't see 'em.

46

calcium (metal)

In Figure 4-18 the right heart border and ascending aorta are not visualized because the pneumonic process is inadequately penetrated. It is possible that these structures don't project to the right of the spine in this patient. The pneumonia is actually in the RLL.

47

The silhouette sign cannot be applied to the right heart border if this border:

(a) ** _____

(b) ** _____

47

(a) overlies the spine

(b) if the film is under-penetrated

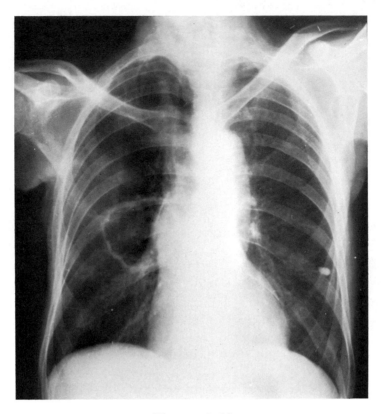

Figure 4-19

48   **48**

To obliterate the cardiovascular border or diaphragm,
lesions must be of _____ density.   water
Calcified lesions and air-filled cavities will not give
a silhouette sign because: They are of different
                                                           roentgen density (not
**   water density).
_____ _____

Figure 4-19 shows an air-filled cavity in contact with the ascending
aorta border. This border is preserved because the lesion in contact
is of different roentgen density than the heart.

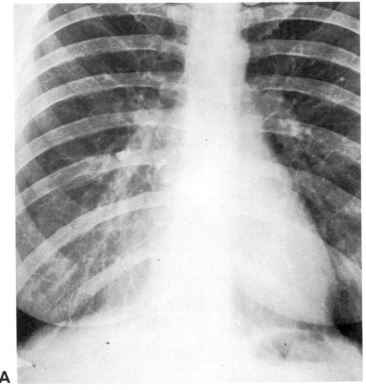

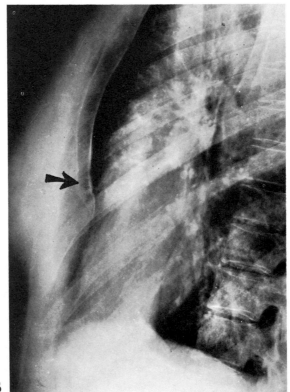

Figure 4-20

49

In some patients with funnel breast (pectus excavatum), the right heart border is obliterated by the water density of the depressed soft tissues of the chest wall. Thus, the silhouette sign (can / cannot) be applied to patients with _____ _____. (Funnel breast seldom occurs in the Italian film colony.)

49

cannot

pectus excavatum
(funnel breast)

Figure 4-20, *A*, gives the appearance of a silhouette sign on the right. Figure 4-20, *B*, the lateral view, shows that a funnel breast deformity is actually the cause of this silhouette sign.

50

A pulmonary vessel or "fat pad" along the pericardium may occasionally obliterate a small part of the heart border. Thus, at times, it is possible for a normal patient to show a _____ _____.

50

silhouette sign

REVIEW

I   I

From the following descriptions of PA films, localize the lesion. Specify the segment, when possible.

(a) An infiltrate in the left lower lung obliterates the left heart border:

_____

(b) An infiltrate obliterates the aortic knob:
   **
_____

(c) A density at the right lung base fails to obliterate the heart:

_____   (a) lingula

(d) A pleural effusion overlaps but does not obliterate the heart border. It is (encapsulated / free) (anteriorly / posteriorly).

(b) apical posterior segment, LUL (#1-3)

(c) RLL

(e) An infiltrate in the left lower lung obliterates the diaphragm:

_____   (d) encapsulated posteriorly

(e) LLL

(f) A localized left pulmonary infiltrate obliterates the descending aorta just below the aortic knob:
   **
_____   (f) superior segment, LLL (#6)

II   **II**

True or False?

(a) A lesion in the anterior segment of the RUL
(#2) will not obliterate the ascending aorta.

_____

(b) A mass in the posterior mediastinum will not
obliterate the heart border. _____

(c) A lesion in the anterior segment of the LLL
(#8) will not obliterate the left heart border.

_____

(d) A lesion in the anterior segment of the LUL
(#2) will not obliterate the aortic knob.

_____

(a) False

(b) True

(c) True

(d) True

The silhouette sign is nearly always an abnormal finding. It may be
present even when you can't see the disease causing it. On every chest
film you see from now on, look for the silhouette sign.

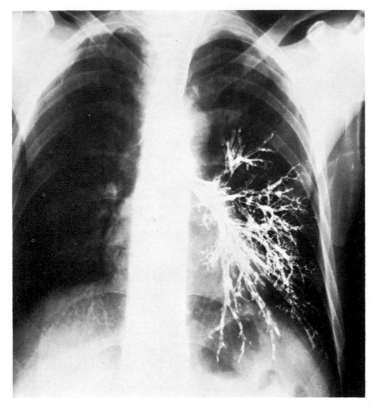

Figure 5–1

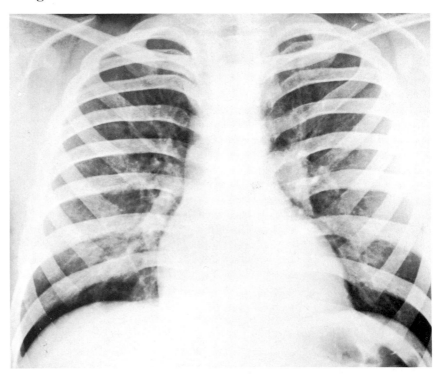

Figure 5–2

Chapter 5

THE AIR BRONCHOGRAM SIGN

1

We do not see the intrapulmonary bronchi on a normal chest roentgenogram. In order to see them we have to instill opaque contrast material (metal density) into their lumens. This roentgen procedure, as you know, is called a _____.

1

bronchogram

Figure 5-1 shows a bronchogram of the left lung. Contrast medium fills the bronchi.

2

The branching linear markings seen in the lungs on plain films are blood vessels, which are water density. Because they contain air, are surrounded by the _____ in the alveoli, and have very thin walls, the _____ are *not* visible on the normal chest roentgenogram.

2

air

bronchi

Figure 5-2 shows a normal chest roentgenogram. The branching markings emanating from the hila are vessels (arteries and veins).

3

In the normal chest the bronchi are surrounded by air in the _____, contain _____, and have _____ walls.

3

alveoli

air

thin

97

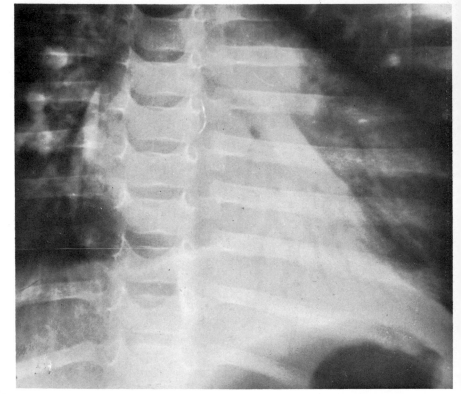

Figure 5-4

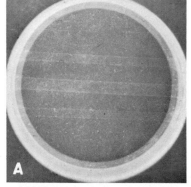

Figure 5-3

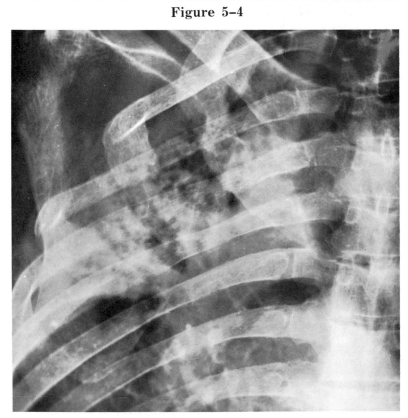

Figure 5-5

4

Now, let's see if you've got the concept. The bronchi are not seen on a normal chest roentgenogram because:

** _____

_____

they have thin walls, they contain air, and they are surrounded by air in the alveoli.

5

What can we do with this concept? Hang on. Visualization of air in the intrapulmonary bronchi on a chest roentgenogram is called the **air bronchogram sign**. The presence of an air bronchogram is (normal / abnormal).

abnormal

6

Now let's try it experimentally. In Figure 5-3, *A*, the situation in the normal lung is portrayed. The straws ("bronchi") are filled with air and surrounded by air. They are barely visible on the roentgenogram. In *B*, the air bronchogram sign is represented. The air-filled straws have been immersed in water and their _____ are clearly seen.

lumens

7

The visualization of air in the bronchi is known as an _____ _____.

air bronchogram

Figures 5-4 and 5-5 illustrate the air bronchogram sign in 2 cases of pneumonia. The bronchi appear as branching black lines. The Bucky film enhances the air bronchogram sign by increasing the contrast (Figure 5-5).

8

Water and gas density are involved in the air bronchogram sign. If an air-filled bronchus is to be seen, it must be surrounded by _____ _____.

water density

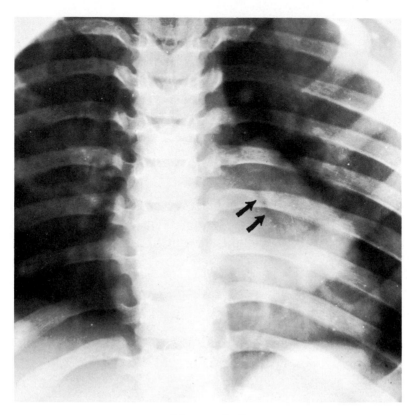

Figure 5–6

9

Air-filled bronchi can be seen if surrounded by pneumonia which, as we know, is _____ density. (Don't you dare miss this one!)

9

water

10

What good is the sign? Well, for one thing, bronchi are pulmonary structures; therefore, visualization of the bronchi denotes a _____ lesion, and excludes a pleural or mediastinal lesion.

10

pulmonary

Figure 5-6 shows a dense area of infiltrate with an air-filled bronchus (arrows) within the lesion. Because there is an air bronchogram sign we know the lesion is in the lung and not in the mediastinum. It was pneumonia.

11

The air bronchogram may be seen in pneumonia, pulmonary edema, pulmonary infarcts, and certain chronic lung lesions. As long as the bronchi are air-filled and the surrounding lung is not, an _____ _____ sign will be present.

11

air bronchogram

12

Do we always see an air bronchogram with pulmonary lesions? Not at all. If the bronchi are filled with secretions or are destroyed, a _____ lesion will not show an air bronchogram.

12

pulmonary

13

In pneumonia, if the bronchi are filled with secretions there (will / will not) be an air bronchogram within the lesion.

13

will not

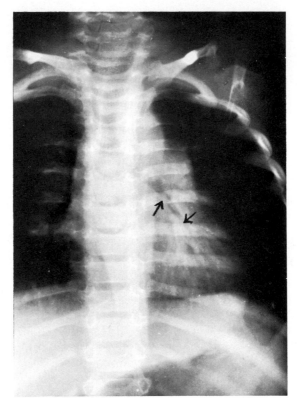

Figure 5-7

14

The air bronchogram denotes a pulmonary lesion. Pleural, mediastinal, and chest wall disease cannot give an air bronchogram sign because they:
** _____

do not contain any bronchi

15

The *absence* of an air bronchogram within a lesion is of little help in localization, since the lesion may then be located either within the _____ or outside the _____.

lung

lung

16

So far it's easy. But remember that a pulmonary lesion may *not* show an air bronchogram because the bronchi may be (*check correct answers*):

(a) destroyed
(b) filled with fluid
(c) congenitally absent

✓(a) destroyed

✓(b) filled with fluid

✓(c) congenitally absent

(There's one born every minute!)

17

Let's wrap up this concept: If the bronchi are seen there must be a _____ lesion. If the bronchi are not seen the lesion could be either _____ or _____.

pulmonary

pulmonary

extrapulmonary (chest wall, pleura, mediastinum)

18

Have a frame on the house: In *infants* and *young children*, the proximal portions of the lobar bronchi often lie within the soft tissues of the mediastinum. Like the trachea, then, they can be seen normally, since they are outlined by the water density of the mediastinum.

Figure 5-7 shows an *infant* in whom the LLL bronchus is visible because it is surrounded by the water density of the mediastinum (arrows). Note the air-filled trachea, seen for the same reason. Remember, this is normal.

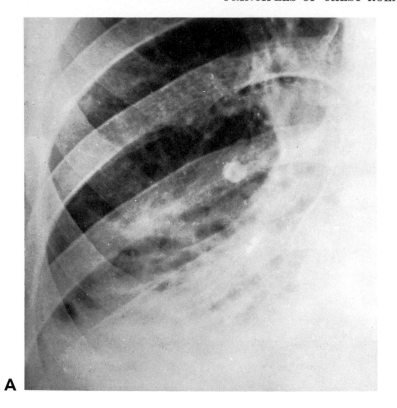

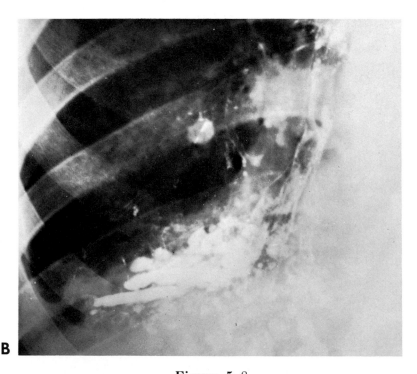

Figure 5–8

19   19

Are there any other uses of the air bronchogram?
Bronchi crowded together denote a collapsed lung
segment or lobe. This can be recognized by bron-
chography, but also is evident on plain films if you   air
see _____ filled bronchi that are
_____ together.   crowded

Figure 5-8, *A*, shows crowded air-filled bronchi in the RML and the
RLL. This indicates collapse of these lobes. Figure 5-8, *B*, is a bronchogram of the same case.

20   20

Here's another example of how the air bronchogram
sign may indicate the type of pulmonary lesion:
Dilated bronchi (in a bronchogram) signify bronchiectasis. Similarly, the visualization on the plain
film of dilated *air-filled* bronchi denotes _____.   bronchiectasis

Look again at Figure 5-8, *A* & *B*:

    collapse

      +

    bronchiectasis

    bronchiectatic collapse

21   21

An astute observer can occasionally identify an air
bronchogram when the pulmonary infiltrate itself is
not apparent, as in a lesion posterior to the left side
of the heart. Thus a disease process in the lung can
be recognized by the _____ _____
alone.   air bronchogram

REVIEW

I

Which of the following conditions may show an air bronchogram?

(a) tuberculosis
(b) empyema
(c) mediastinal bronchogenic cyst
(d) staphylococcal pneumonia
(e) lipoma of the chest wall
(f) pulmonary edema

I

(a) tuberculosis

(d) staphyloccal pneumonia

(f) pulmonary edema

For those who have answered this incorrectly, we would like to point out once again that pleural, mediastinal, or chest wall lesions cannot show an air bronchogram because there are no bronchi in these sites.

II

Recognition of an air bronchogram on the chest film tells you that the lesion is in the _____.
If the bronchi are crowded together, it indicates _____ ; and if they are dilated, _____ is present. If you see an air bronchogram, there must be _____ disease even if you can't see the disease itself.

II

lung

collapse

bronchiectasis

pulmonary

Chapter 6

LOBAR AND SEGMENTAL COLLAPSE

We are now going to apply the roentgen anatomy you learned in Chapters 2 and 3 to the subject of pulmonary collapse. But first we'd better define a few terms.

1

A lung, a lobe, or a segment under certain abnormal conditions may be increased or decreased in size. *Collapse* obviously refers to a _____ in the volume of a lung, lobe, or segment.

1

decrease

> Henceforth, we will deal only with lobar and segmental collapse, but most of the information to be presented applies equally well to collapse of the whole lung.

2

We use the term *collapse* to refer to a lobe or segment whose _____ is diminished.

2

volume

> The word *atelectasis* is often used synonymously with collapse and is widely accepted. But atelectasis means different things to different people, so we deleted it from our dictionary. Guts we've got.

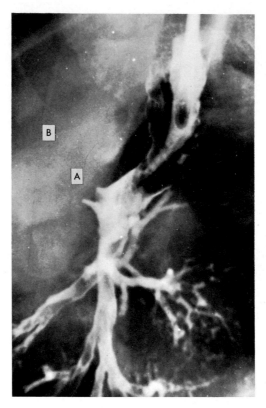

Figure 6–1

3

Obstruction, *compression*, and *contraction* are the 3 mechanisms that cause collapse. Now, again, collapse refers to a _____ in _____ of a lobe or segment.

decrease

volume

4

Obstruction is the most common cause of collapse. This obstruction may be *central*, i.e., a single lesion blocking a lobar or segmental bronchus; or *peripheral*, in which case there are myriads of small plugs which _____ many of the smaller bronchi.

obstruct (block)

5

In obstructive collapse, air cannot enter the alveoli distal to the obstruction. The alveolar air already present is absorbed, and the corresponding lobe or segment ultimately _____ in volume, or collapses.

decreases

6

The central form of collapse, which results from _____ of a lobar or segmental bronchus, is caused by either an *intrinsic* or *extrinsic* lesion.

obstruction

7

Central intrinsic obstruction is most commonly caused by bronchogenic carcinoma. Foreign body and inflammatory bronchial disease (e.g., bronchial tuberculosis) are other important causes of central _____ obstructive collapse.

intrinsic

Figure 6-1 is a bronchogram showing a central intrinsic obstructing carcinoma (A) in the RUL bronchus, causing collapse of the RUL (B).

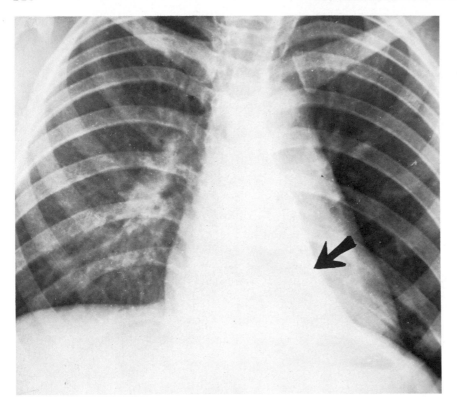

Figure 6-2

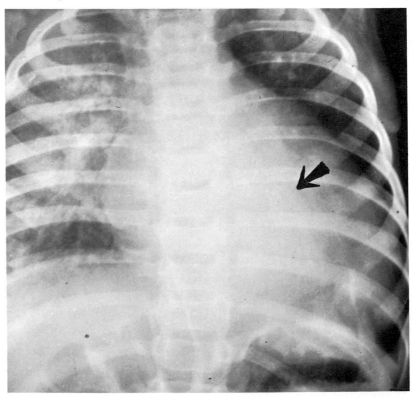

Figure 6-3

8

8

Masses, such as enlarged lymph nodes, mediastinal tumor, aneurysm, or even a big heart, may compress a lobar or segmental bronchus from without, causing central collapse by _____ pressure.

extrinsic

Figure 6-2 is an obvious case of LLL collapse (arrow). Figure 6-3 is more subtle, but shows collapse (arrow) caused by an enlarged heart. The triangular density is rather typical of LLL collapse.

9

9

As a result of inflammatory exudate, mucus, etc., many of the smaller bronchi may become plugged, resulting in (central / peripheral) obstructive collapse.

peripheral

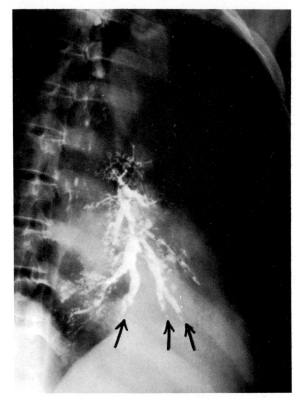

Figure 6–4

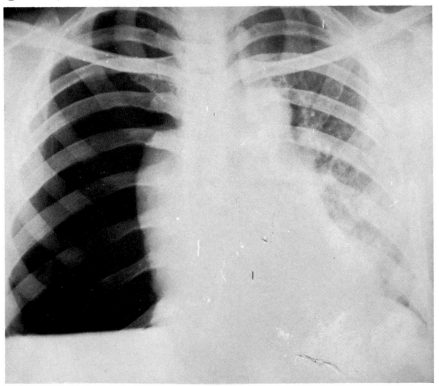

Figure 6–5

10   **10**

Peripheral obstructive collapse is commonly seen in
pneumonia and after operation.   It often clears
spontaneously as the plugs are absorbed or coughed
up. Figure 6-4 is a case of LLL collapse due to
multiple peripheral plugs resulting from pneumonia.
The bronchogram shows many _____
bronchi (arrows).   obstructed (plugged)

11   **11**

As we stated earlier, compression, contraction, and
_____ are the 3 mechanisms which
cause collapse, the latter being the most important.   obstruction
A pneumothorax or pleural effusion squeezes air from
the lung and causes collapse by _____.   compression

Figure 6-5 shows marked compression collapse of the entire right lung
from pneumothorax. There is an air-fluid level in the right pleural
cavity.

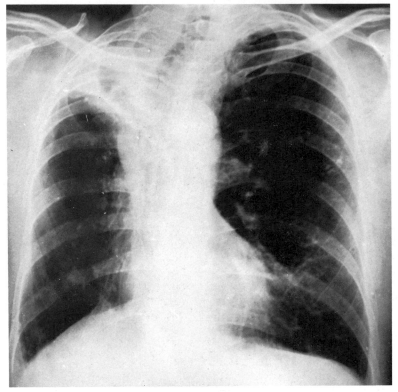

Figure 6-6

12   12

In chronic tuberculosis or pulmonary fibrosis from
any cause, e.g., silicosis, scarring may result in diminution in volume. This represents collapse from
_____.   contraction

Figure 6-6 is a case of contraction collapse of the RUL secondary to
tuberculosis.

13   13

Don't get the idea that obstruction invariably causes
collapse. Occasionally, distal to an obstruction, a
large amount of inflammatory secretions or edema
accumulates, preventing diminution in size. In this
situation there is _____ without
collapse.   obstruction

The radiologic jargon for this is "drowned lung." In this condition the
obstructed lobe or segment may actually be enlarged.

14   14

Here's a summary frame: The 3 mechanisms for   obstruction
collapse are _____, _____, and   compression
_____.   contraction

(a) Bronchogenic carcinoma is an (intrinsic / ex-   (a) intrinsic
    trinsic) (central / peripheral) cause of   central
    (contraction / obstruction) collapse.   obstruction

(b) Aneurysm is an (intrinsic / extrinsic) cause of (b) extrinsic
    (central / peripheral) (compression / obstruc-   central
    tion) collapse.   obstruction

(c) Pneumonia is a cause of (central / peripheral)   (c) peripheral
    (compression / obstruction) collapse.   obstruction

15

List 2 causes for each of the following.

(a) central intrinsic obstruction collapse:
**
_____

(b) central extrinsic obstruction collapse:
**
_____

(c) peripheral obstruction collapse:
**
_____

(d) compression collapse:
**
_____

(e) contraction collapse:
**
_____

15

(a) bronchogenic carcinoma, foreign body, inflammatory disease of bronchus

(b) enlarged lymph nodes, large heart, aneurysm, mediastinal tumor

(c) postoperative, pneumonia

(d) pneumothorax, pleural effusion

(e) tuberculosis, silicosis, pulmonary fibrosis from other cause

These are not the only ones. Give yourself credit for any logical answer, such as metastatic fecalith.

16

It's easy to recognize compression collapse by seeing the pneumothorax or the pleural fluid causing it. In contraction collapse, irregular scarring in the collapsed segment is usually evident. But obstruction collapse is often more difficult to diagnose. All the roentgen signs, direct and indirect, are based on diminished _____ of the affected lobe or segment.

16

volume

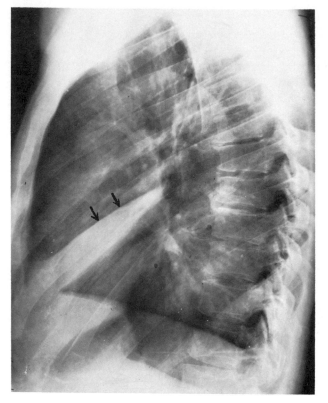

Figure 6–7

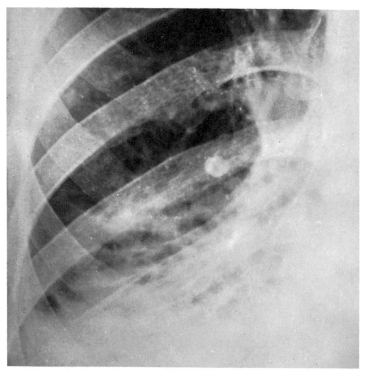

Figure 6–8

17

If the volume of a lobe or segment is diminished (collapse), the septa bounding it, when visible, will be displaced. The displacement is, of course, in the direction of the collapsed lung. The most reliable direct roentgen sign of collapse, therefore, is _____ of the interlobar _____ bounding the affected part of the lung.

displacement

septa (fissures)

Figure 6-7 is a lateral view that shows the minor fissure (arrows) displaced downward in RML collapse.

18

18

When a lobe or segment collapses, it loses aeration, and the affected lung becomes (more / less) radiopaque. This is a *second* direct sign of collapse. Hold on, though! This sign *by itself* does not indicate collapse. Almost any disease process, with or without collapse, may show _____ radiopacity.

more

increased

Figure 6-7 also shows the increased density of the collapsed RML.

19

19

If a lobe or segment is diminished in volume but still contains some air, the vascular markings within it will be visible and crowded into a smaller space. If the bronchi within the collapsed area are visible (the _____ _____ sign) they, too, will appear _____ together. This vascular or bronchial finding represents the *third* direct sign of collapse.

air bronchogram (remember?)

crowded

Figure 6-8 is a case of RML and RLL collapse showing visible bronchi crowded together.

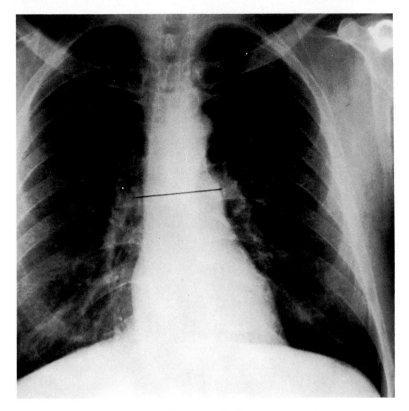

Figure 6–9

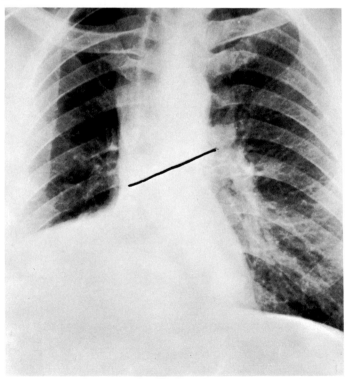

Figure 6–10

20

The 3 direct signs of collapse, then, are:

  (1) ** _____

  (2) ** _____

  (3) ** _____

Indicate by a check mark which of these signs is the most reliable.

20

✓ (1) displaced septa

   (2) increased radiopacity

   (3) vascular or bronchial crowding

21

There are various *indirect* signs of collapse, the most reliable of which is hilar displacement. This is the only _____ sign which, by itself, always indicates collapse.

21

indirect

22

To appreciate hilar displacement one must, of course, know the relative positions of the normal hila. In over 97 per cent of normal individuals the left hilum is slightly higher than the right. In the remaining 3 per cent the hila are at the same level.* Thus, if the left hilum is lower than the right, this is (normal / abnormal) and indicates _____.

22

abnormal

collapse (LLL, of course)

Figure 6-9 shows the normal relationship of the hila (line). Figure 6-10 shows downward and medial displacement of the right hilum in postoperative collapse of the RML and RLL.

---

* The figures cited are based on 1000 normal chest roentgenograms studied by one of us with nothing better to do.

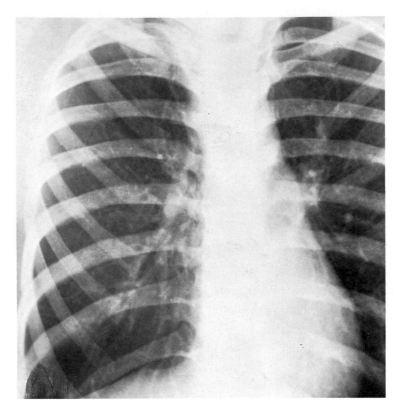

Figure 6–11

23   **23**

A collapsed lobe will usually displace the hilum on
that side. The displacement will be in the direction
of the collapse. Thus, in collapse of the RUL the
right hilum will be (depressed / elevated).   elevated

Figure 6-11 shows upward displacement of the right hilum in RUL
collapse. Follow the right pulmonary artery branches to their con-
vergence. This is the hilum. The RUL is so markedly collapsed that
it is barely visible in the apex of the thorax.

24   **24**

In collapse of the LLL, the left hilum will be
(depressed / elevated).   depressed

25   **25**

We said that collapse "usually" causes hilar displacement. Owing to its small size and somewhat central
position, RML collapse seldom causes displacement
of the right hilum. The same principle applies to   If you said *lingula*,
another portion of the lung. Guess which: _____.   you're right.

If you didn't, don't feel bad. Some of the radiology residents who
tested this program didn't know either. They do now.

26   **26**

The other indirect signs are based on the concept of
replacement of the space created when collapse
occurs. For instance, in lower lobe collapse the diaphragm will often be (elevated / depressed). This is
a second indirect sign of collapse.   elevated

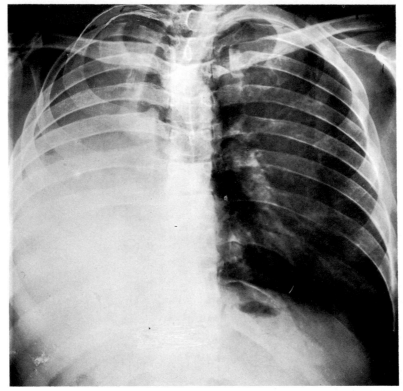

Figure 6-12

27

Similarly, in LUL collapse the trachea shifts from its normal midline position toward the (left / right) to help fill the vacated space.

Tracheal shift is infrequent in collapse of the middle lobe, lingula, or lower lobes because these areas are some distance from the trachea.

left

28

In marked collapse of one or more lobes the heart and mediastinum may shift (away from / toward) the side of collapse.

Shift of any of the mediastinal structures constitutes another indirect sign of collapse.

toward

Figure 6-12 shows marked shift of the trachea and heart to the right, as a result of collapse of the entire right lung. Believe it or not, this was the result of a fractured right bronchus.

29

At this point we have learned 3 indirect signs of collapse. These are:

(1) ** _____
(2) ** _____
(3) ** _____

(1) hilar displacement

(2) elevation of diaphragm

(3) shift of mediastinal structures

30

An indirect sign difficult to recognize and to evaluate is the change in the size of the rib cage on the affected side. To compensate for the _____ volume, the ribs lie (closer together / farther apart).

decreased

closer together

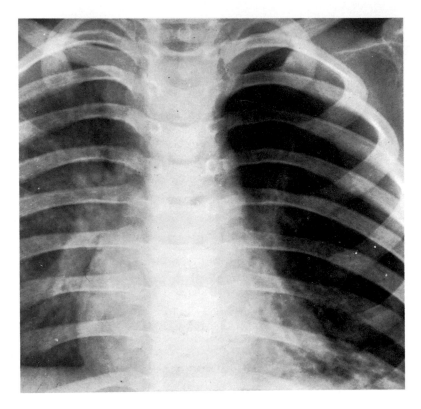

Figure 6–13

31

Finally, the normal lung adjacent to the collapsed portion may overexpand to fill the vacated space. This is known as compensatory emphysema, and is recognized by (increased / decreased) lucency.

31

increased

Figure 6-13 shows compensatory emphysema of the LUL resulting from LLL collapse.

32

As the lung adjacent to an area of collapse expands, the vascular markings in it spread apart. This contributes to the increased blackness of the lung in _____ emphysema.

32

compensatory

33

The degree of collapse is variable, and depends on the amount of edema and pneumonia distal to the obstruction. Obviously, the more edema or pneumonia, the (greater / less) will be the signs of collapse.

33

less

34

Let's take a breather. The most reliable indirect sign of collapse is _____ _____.
What is the most reliable direct sign of collapse:

    ** _____

While you're at it, what are the other direct signs:

    ** _____
    ** _____

34

hilar displacement

displacement of the fissures

increased radiopacity

crowding of the bronchial or vascular markings

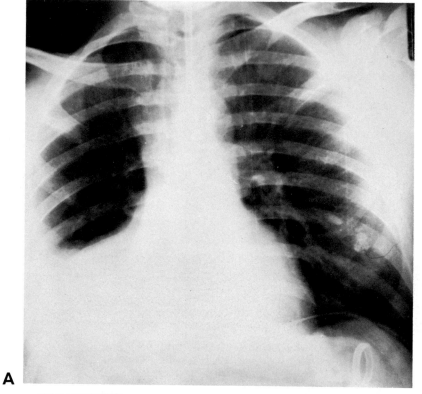

A

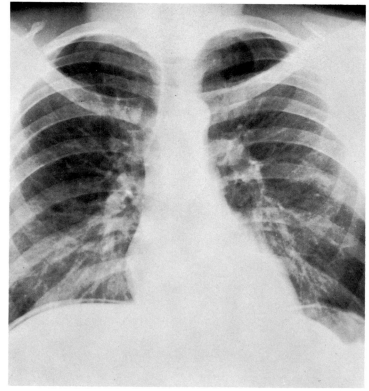

B

Figure 6–14

35

Try your newly acquired skill on the following case. Figure 6-14, *A*, is a film taken on a hospital patient who suddenly developed shortness of breath and fever. Figure 6-14, *B*, is a film taken several hours later.

(a) Which lobes are collapsed:
   **
   _____ _____

(b) List the *direct* signs which led you to this diagnosis:
   **
   _____

(c) List the *indirect* signs which aided in the diagnosis:
   **
   _____

(d) What is the most likely etiology of the collapse:
   **
   _____

35

(a) RML and RLL

(b) 1. displacement of minor fissure
   2. radiopacity of the collapsed lobes

(c) 1. downward shift of the right hilum
   2. shift of trachea
   3. compensatory emphysema of RUL

(d) Postoperative. This has produced peripheral obstruction secondary to mucus plugs. Note the free air beneath the right diaphragm (from a laparotomy).

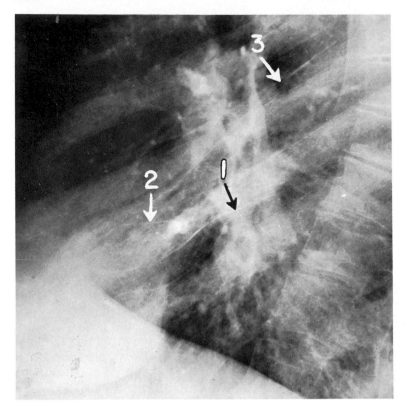

Figure 6–15

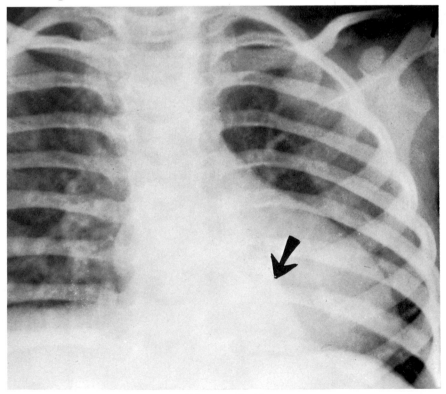

Figure 6–16

36   **36**

Now for the roentgen appearance of collapse of each
lobe. The RLL and LLL (and corresponding major
fissures) collapse posteriorly, medially, and downward.
Thus, in the lateral view, the major septum is dis-   backward
placed (forward / backward) and (upward / down-
ward).   downward

The medial shift can be recognized only in the frontal view. Figure
6-15 is a lateral view showing shift of the right major fissure (1)
backward and downward in RLL collapse.   Compare it to the normal
position of the left major fissure (3). The minor fissure (2) is also
depressed.

37   **37**

In fairly marked collapse of a lower lobe, the frontal view may show (medial / lateral) displacement
of the major fissure.   This is recognized as the
outer boundary of a triangular shadow of opacity
adjacent to the spine.   medial

Figure 6-16 shows a triangular area of increased density through the
heart shadow, representing LLL collapse (arrow).

38   **38**

On the frontal projection, RML collapse is often indicated by (upward / downward) displacement of the
minor fissure.   downward

39   **39**

Because of their smaller size, the collapsed RML
and lingula often cast only a faint shadow in the
frontal projection, and the minor fissure displacement
may not be apparent.   The silhouette sign may then
come to the rescue.   Collapse of the entire RML
obliterates the _____ heart border,
and collapse of the lingula obliterates the _____   right
_____ _____.   The loss of the cardiac sil-
houette may then be the only sign of the disease.   left heart border

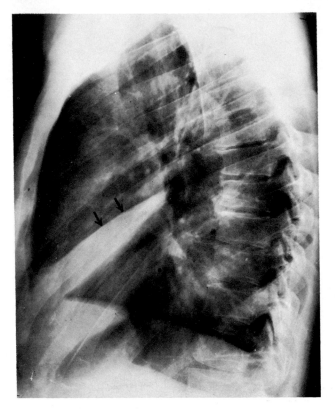

Figure 6–17

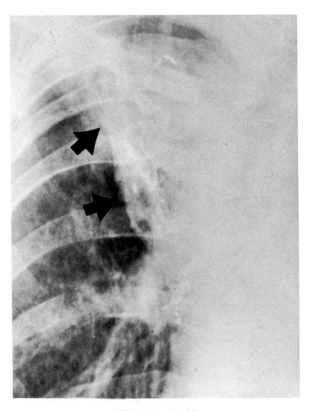

Figure 6–18

40

On the lateral view, RML collapse is indicated if
the _____ fissure and lower half of
the _____ fissure are seen closer
together.

40

minor

major

> Figure 6-17 is a lateral view of RML collapse, showing the minor
> (arrows) and major fissures closer together than normal.

41

The collapsed RUL is displaced upward, medially,
and anteriorly. On the frontal view, the minor fissure reflects this by being displaced (upward /
downward) and (medially / laterally).

41

upward

medially

> Figure 6-18 shows RUL collapse with elevation and medial displacement
> of the minor fissure (arrows).

42

The RUL may collapse so completely that it blends
with the superior mediastinum. In this case, the
direct signs of collapse may be absent in the frontal
view. What important indirect sign might alert you
to the presence of RUL collapse?

42

** _____

right hilar elevation

43

In RUL collapse the lateral view shows (upward /
downward) shift of the minor fissure. The upper
part of the major fissure will be shifted (posteriorly
/ anteriorly).

43

upward

anteriorly

44

The LUL collapses in a manner similar to the RUL,
namely, medially, _____, and _____.

44

upward

anteriorly

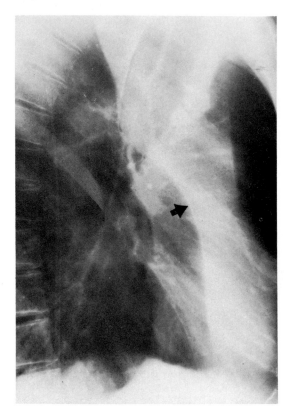

Figure 6-19

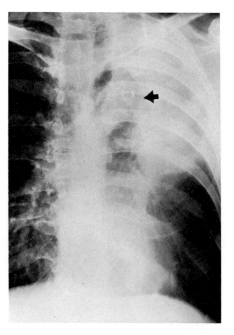

Figure 6-20

45   **45**

In collapse of the LUL, on the lateral view the
major fissure will be displaced (forward / backward).   forward

> Figure 6-19 is a lateral view showing typical LUL collapse with anterior
> shift and bowing of the major fissure (arrow).

46   **46**

If only a single segment is collapsed, the direct signs,
minimal in degree, can usually be recognized; but
the indirect signs are generally absent. It is hardly
ever possible to diagnose *subsegmental* collapse from
plain films because the overall decrease in _____
is so small.   volume

47   **47**

Afterthought: Collapse of a whole lung often produces
an additional indirect sign — herniation of the
normal lung into the involved thorax. This sign may
occur with (mild / marked) collapse of a single lobe.   marked

> Figure 6-20 shows herniation of the right lung (arrow) across the
> midline in collapse of the LUL. This is the same case as Figure 6-19,
> which shows the herniated lung anterior to the heart and aorta.

REVIEW

I

A. List the 3 mechanisms that produce lobar or segmental collapse:

(1) _____
(2) _____
(3) _____

B. Which of these mechanisms are involved in collapse from

(1) pleural effusion: _____
(2) silicosis: _____
(3) aneurysm: _____

I

A

(1) obstruction
(2) compression
(3) contraction

B

(1) compression
(2) contraction
(3) obstruction

II

A. Which of the following causes of obstruction collapse are intrinsic and which are extrinsic?

(1) foreign body: _____
(2) enlarged heart: _____
(3) enlarged lymph nodes: _____
(4) bronchogenic carcinoma: _____

B. Which of the following causes of obstruction collapse are central and which are peripheral?

(1) mediastinal tumor: _____
(2) inflammatory stricture: _____
(3) pneumonia: _____

II

A

(1) intrinsic
(2) extrinsic
(3) extrinsic
(4) intrinsic

B

(1) central
(2) central
(3) peripheral

III

A. List the 3 *direct* roentgen signs of collapse:

  (1) ** _____

  (2) ** _____

  (3) ** _____

B. List 4 of the *indirect* roentgen signs of collapse:

  (1) ** _____

  (2) ** _____

  (3) ** _____

  (4) ** _____

III

A

  (1) displacement of septa

  (2) increased radiopacity

  (3) vascular or bronchial crowding

B

  (1) hilar displacement

  (2) elevation of diaphragm

  (3) shift of mediastinal structures

  (4) compensatory emphysema

  (5) narrowing of rib cage

  (6) herniation

Chapter 7 | THE PLEURA

1   1

The periphery of the base of each pleural cavity forms a rather deep sulcus around the dome of the corresponding hemidiaphragm. This is called the costophrenic sinus or angle. The deepest and most caudal portion of the _____ angle is its posterior section.

costophrenic

We prefer the word *angle* over *sulcus* or *sinus*.

2   2

The costophrenic angle has 4 sections: the anterior, posterior, medial, and lateral. The deepest, most caudal portion is the _____ costophrenic angle. The lateral _____ angle is also fairly deep.

posterior

costophrenic

3   3

The posterior costophrenic angle is not visible on the PA teleo film because the dome of the corresponding hemidiaphragm extends (above / below) it.

above

This angle is, however, well shown in the lateral view.

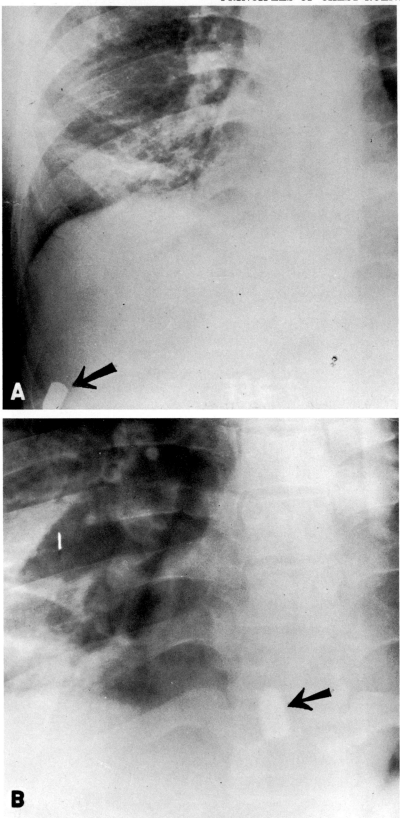

Figure 7-1

4   4

The Lothario whose films are shown in Figure 7-1
slammed the back door just as the husband fired.
The bullet that hit the fleeing lover was almost
spent, merely penetrating his chest wall and dropping
harmlessly into the pleural space. Figure 7-1 illustrates the depth of the _____ costo-
phrenic angle as well as the hazards of sex.   posterior

> *A*, Upright film. The bullet (arrow) in the posterior costophrenic angle
>   appears to lie in the abdomen.
> *B*, Recumbent film. The bullet has shifted to the medial costophrenic
>   angle.

5   5

Free pleural fluid, whether it be blood, lymph, exudate, or transudate, is heavier than the air-filled
lung and sinks to the base of the pleural cavity in
the _____ position.   upright

6   6

On the upright film, free pleural fluid often causes
the normally deep _____ and lateral
costophrenic angles to appear shallow or obliterated.   posterior

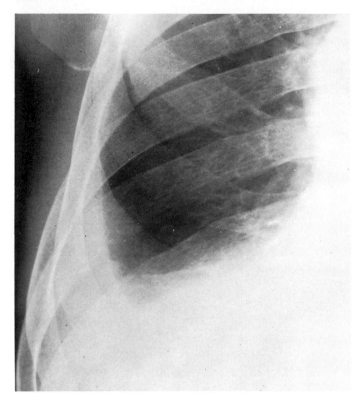

Figure 7-2

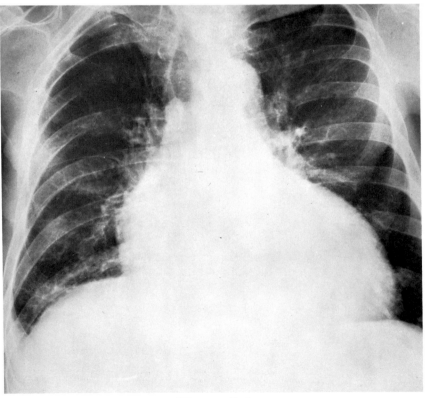

Figure 7-3

7   7

Free fluid often presents a concave upper border,
or *meniscus*, which appears to extend higher
_____ than medially, as shown in Figure 7-2.   laterally

8   8

In the upright position, free fluid may become trap-
ped between the under surface of the lung and the
top of the hemidiaphragm. The resultant roentgen
shadow strikingly resembles an elevated hemidiaphragm. Thus, instead of the curved _____
pattern, we may have a *subpulmonary* pattern.   meniscus

In Figure 7-3, what appears to be an elevated right hemidiaphragm is
actually subpulmonary fluid. The true diaphragm lies in normal position
but is obscured by the parallel layer of free fluid. We'll prove this
with a decubitus view in a few minutes.

9   9

The subpulmonary pattern is more common with
smaller amounts of fluid, the meniscus pattern with
larger amounts of fluid. Subpulmonary fluid lies   lung
beneath the _____ and above the
_____.   diaphragm

Remember, now, these patterns are seen only in the upright position.

10   **10**

The two common patterns of free pleural fluid seen   meniscus
on the PA teleo film are the _____ and
_____ patterns.   subpulmonary

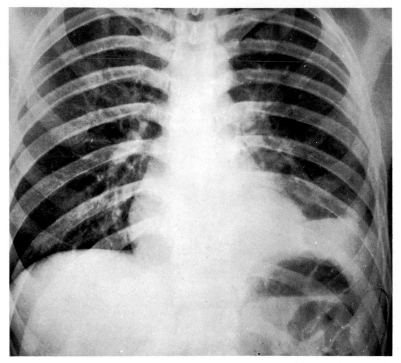

Figure 7–4

11

We are now faced with the practical problem of recognizing subpulmonary fluid, since it so closely simulates an elevated _____ on the PA and lateral teleo films.

11

hemidiaphragm

12

Normally the gastric air bubble often hugs the dome of the left hemidiaphragm. With left subpulmonary fluid, the gas bubble may lie (farther than normal from / closer than normal to) the spurious "diaphragm."

12

farther than
    normal from

Figure 7-4 shows a left subpulmonary effusion separating the gas bubble from the simulated diaphragm.
One problem, though: In some healthy individuals, the gas bubble *normally* is separated from the diaphragm in the frontal view.

13

The subpulmonary fluid tends to fill the costophrenic angles, so they are often (deeper / shallower) than normal.

13

shallower

14

List 3 signs which should alert you to the presence of subpulmonary fluid on the upright films:

    (1) ** _____
    (2) ** _____
    (3) ** _____

14

(1) high "diaphragm"

(2) separation of stomach bubble from "diaphragm"

(3) shallow costophrenic angles

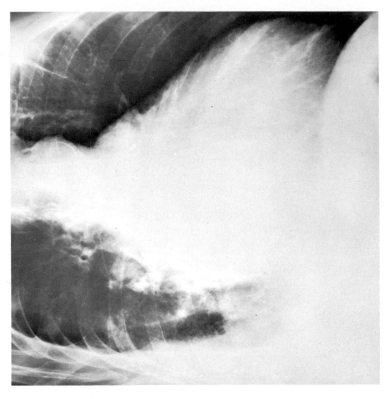

Figure 7–5

15   15

Gravitational views are essential for confirming the
presence of subpulmonary fluid. Which one would
you recommend for this purpose?

** _____   lateral decubitus view

> Of course, the affected side should be dependent.
> Figure 7-5 is a right lateral decubitus view of the patient shown in
> Figure 7-3. The free fluid has gravitated to the dependent side of the
> right pleural cavity.

16   16

The AP supine view will also reveal the presence of
free fluid.   In this position the fluid gravitates   posteriorly
(anteriorly / posteriorly) and causes the affected
hemithorax to appear (more / less) radiolucent.   less

> However, the lateral decubitus view will reveal smaller amounts of fluid.

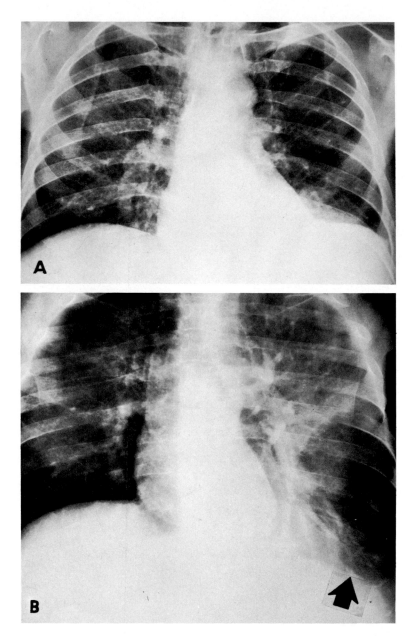

Figure 7–6

17   17

In Figure 7-6, the PA teleo film, *A*, shows 2 signs
of subpulmonary fluid:

   (1) ** _____

   (2) ** _____

                                               (1) shallow costophrenic

The AP supine view, *B*, shows the left hemidia-   angle
phragm (arrow) in normal position and a haze (fluid)
over the left thorax.   (2) high "diaphragm"

Play it cozy. If either hemidiaphragm appears elevated, order a lateral
decubitus view to exclude subpulmonary effusion.

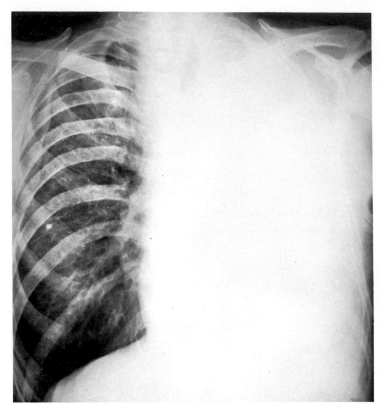

Figure 7–7

18

A fairly large amount of fluid must be present before the heart and mediastinal structures shift toward the opposite thorax. Can you think of a situation in which a *very* large amount of free fluid is present but the mediastinal structures shift *toward* the side of the fluid, as in Figure 7-7?

** _____

18

If you said *obstructive collapse*, you're right. And if you said *collapse due to bronchogenic carcinoma*, you're even righter, since it is the most frequent cause of this combination. The fluid usually results from pleural metastases.
That's what the patient in Figure 7-7 had.

19

In congestive heart failure, free pleural effusion is common. If the fluid is unilateral, it is nearly always on the right side. If the effusion is bilateral, it is almost always larger on the right. We looked up the explanation for this, but drew a _____.

19

20

A patient has a pleural effusion confined to the left hemithorax. Which of the following diagnoses can you exclude?

   (a) tuberculous pleuritis
   (b) pulmonary infarction
   (c) congestive heart failure
   (d) pleural metastases

20

   (c) congestive heart failure

21

Summary time and the answers are easy:

(1) Free pleural fluid usually assumes the _____ pattern or the _____ pattern.

(2) If free fluid is suspected on an upright film, what additional view should be obtained?

_____ _____

(3) If the heart and mediastinum are shifted toward the side of a pleural effusion, what diagnosis is suggested?

_____ _____

(4) Left pleural effusion is rarely caused by:
** _____

21

(1) meniscus
    subpulmonary

(2) lateral decubitus

(3) bronchogenic
    carcinoma (obstruc-
    tion collapse)

(4) congestive heart
    failure

22

Encapsulated (loculated) pleural effusion is attributable to pleural adhesions, pre-existing or developing after the appearance of free fluid.
  Are gravitational views useful in the diagnosis of encapsulated effusion? _____

22

Yes

We meant to trick you. If the fluid *doesn't* shift, it is encapsulated—so the gravitational view *is* useful.

23

Because it is of water density and remains in the same location in all positions, encapsulated fluid may closely resemble pulmonary disease. If an air bronchogram is seen within the lesion (pulmonary disease / encapsulated fluid) can be ruled out.

23

encapsulated fluid

24

We now have 2 signs of encapsulated fluid:

(1) failure to shift with change in position
(2) ** _____

24

absence of air
bronchogram

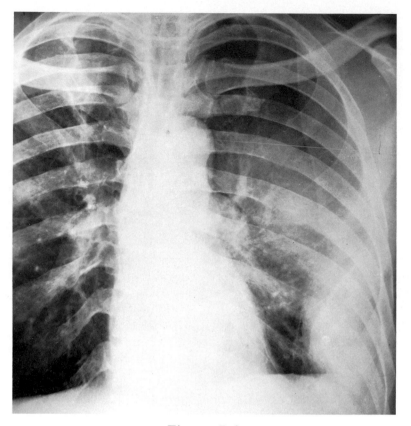

Figure 7–8

25

Consult Figure 7-8, an example of encapsulated fluid in the lower left thorax. The borders of an encapsulation are generally (more / less) convex than those outlining a collapsed or consolidated lobe.

25

more

26

Pleural thickening elsewhere in the same hemithorax is a fourth sign of encapsulated fluid. What's that third sign again?

** _____

26

convex border

27

Name at least 3 roentgen signs of encapsulated pleural fluid:

(1) ** _____
(2) ** _____
(3) ** _____
(4) ** _____

27

(1) failure to shift with change in position

(2) absence of an air bronchogram

(3) convex border

(4) pleural thickening elsewhere in the same hemithorax

28

If the general pleural cavity is obliterated by adhesions, pleural fluid may become _____ in an interlobar fissure.

28

encapsulated

Interlobar encapsulation is most commonly encountered in congestive heart failure.

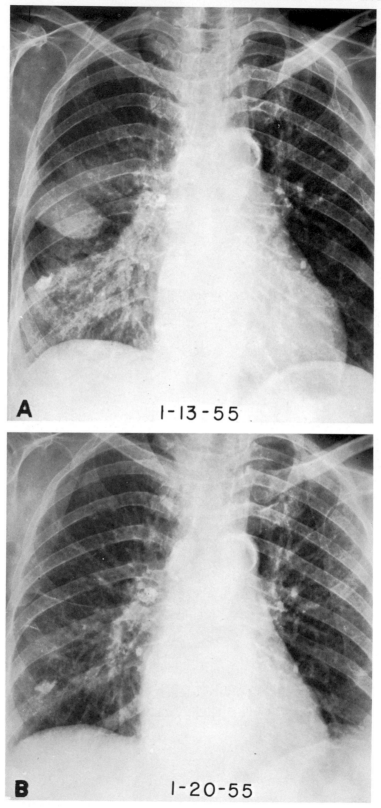

Figure 7–9

29   29

In congestive heart failure, free or encapsulated
pleural fluid disappears rapidly as cardiac compensa-
tion is restored. Figure 7-9, *A*, shows a patient in
congestive failure. Note the tumor-like density in
the right mid-thorax. After successful treatment,
the oval shadow disappeared (*B*).
    What was the shadow in Figure 7-9, *A*?

**
_____
    Exactly where was it?   encapsulated fluid

**
_____   minor fissure

This sequence is fairly common and, in sophisticated circles, has been
termed *vanishing tumor*.

30   30

Encapsulated interlobar effusion is bounded by visceral pleura, and its margins appear (sharp / hazy)
when seen in profile.   sharp

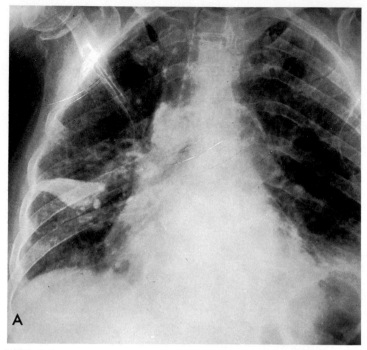

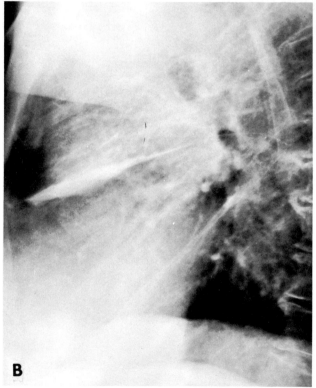

Figure 7-10

31   31

In Figure 7-10, an example of fluid encapsulated in
the minor fissure, the margins of the loculation
appear sharp in the:

(a) PA view
(b) lateral view
(c) both PA and lateral views   (c) both PA and lateral
(d) neither view   views

You will certainly recall that the x-ray beam is usually parallel to this
fissure in both PA and lateral views.

A

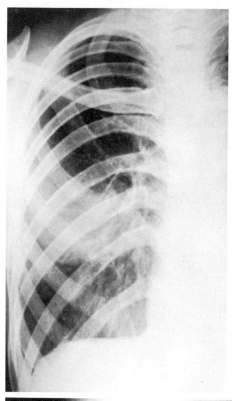

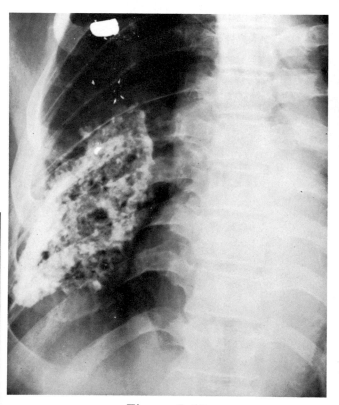

Figure 7–12

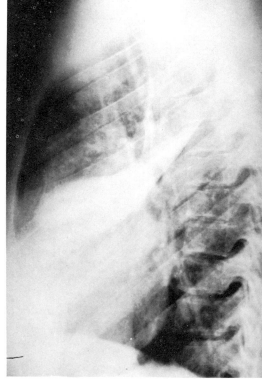

B

Figure 7–11

32

The margins of an encapsulated effusion in the major fissure are sharp in the:
- (a) PA view
- (b) lateral view
- (c) both PA and lateral views
- (d) neither view

32

(b) lateral view

The x-ray beam is parallel to the major fissure only in the lateral view. Figure 7-11, *A & B*, is an example of encapsulated effusion in the major fissure.

33

Pleural thickening without effusion is usually a sign of past disease, now inactive. It is encountered in about 1 per cent of normal adults.
It is indicated by:

- (1) thickening of the pleura around the periphery of the lung
- (2) thickening of the interlobar septa
- (3) partial or complete _____ of the costophrenic angle

33

obliteration

34

Can you think of a roentgen density associated with pleural disease, other than water density and bullets?

** _____

34

actually there are 2:
- (1) gas (pneumothorax)
- (2) calcium

Pneumothorax has already been discussed in previous chapters.

35

Figure 7-12 shows extensive pleural calcification, an occasional finding. It is the result of empyema, pleural effusion, or hemothorax that occurred (months / years) ago. Small calcified pleural plaques occur in certain of the pneumoconioses. What was the cause in this case? ** _____

35

years

gunshot. Another Cincinnati Don Juan.

REVIEW

A. What are the 2 patterns seen with *free* pleural effusions?

  (1) _____

  (2) _____

(1) meniscus
(2) subpulmonary

B. If pleural effusion is confined to the left thorax, what diagnosis usually can be excluded?

  ** _____

congestive heart failure

C. What 3 signs on an upright film should alert you to the presence of fluid between the lung and diaphragm?

  (1) ** _____

  (2) ** _____

  (3) ** _____

(1) high "hemidia-phragm"
(2) separation of stomach bubble from hemidiaphragm
(3) shallow costophrenic angles

D. List 3 signs of encapsulated pleural fluid:

  (1) ** _____

  (2) ** _____

  (3) ** _____

(1) failure to shift with change in position
(2) absence of an air bronchogram
(3) convex border
(4) pleural thickening elsewhere in same hemithorax

Chapter 8

THE EXTRAPLEURAL SPACE

1

1

The pleural cavity lies between the _____ and parietal layers of pleura. The *extrapleural space* surrounds the pleural cavity. It lies between the rib cage and the _____ ____pleura.

visceral

parietal

2

2

The space that lies between the rib cage and parietal pleura is known as the _____ _____.
It is a *potential* space, since the parietal pleura is somewhat adherent to the endothoracic fascia.

extrapleural space

3

3

Lesions that arise in structures within or bordering the extrapleural space may extend into it. The ribs are the most common source of extrapleural lesions.
(True / False)

True

Our experience indicates that rib metastasis is by far the commonest extrapleural lesion.

4

In addition to the _____, the soft
tissues in the extrapleural space and adjacent intercostal region may give rise to extrapleural lesions.
The soft tissues include connective tissue, muscle,
nerves, and vessels.

5

Lesions in the lung or pleura occasionally extend
through the parietal pleura into the extrapleural
space. There are, then, 3 sites of origin of
extrapleural lesions:

(1) _____ _____
(2) _____ _____
(3) lung or pleura

6

List the 3 sources of extrapleural lesions and circle
the most common one:

(1) _____
(2) _____
(3) _____

7

A variety of diseases may involve the extrapleural
space. These include neoplasm, infection (especially
tuberculosis and fungus), and hematoma. Metastatic
neoplasm is the commonest. Metastatic to what?

_____

8

The extrapleural space is most frequently involved
by:

(1) _____
(2) _____
(3) hematoma

4

ribs

5

(1) rib

(2) soft tissues

6

((1) rib)

(2) soft tissues

(3) lung or pleura

7

rib

8

(1) neoplasm

(2) infection

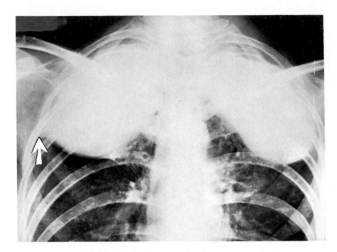

Figure 8–1

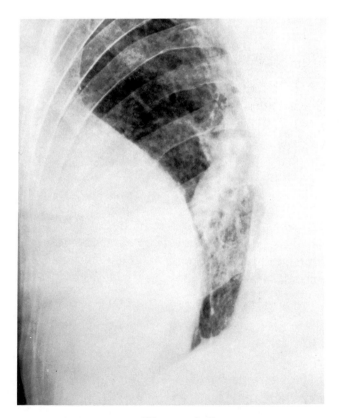

Figure 8–2

9   9

A lesion in the extrapleural space often produces a
characteristic roentgen appearance. Because of the
intact layers of parietal and visceral pleura overlying
it, an extrapleural lesion will often present a very
(sharp / hazy) contour facing the lung.   sharp

The patient shown in Figure 8-1 appears to have internal bosoms or
undescended testes. Nothing so exotic, though. The weird appearance
is the result of mineral oil introduced on purpose into the extrapleural
space. This was formerly used as collapse therapy for pulmonary tuberculosis.
    Note the very sharp margin of this iatrogenic lesion. Your attention
is also called to the tapering edges (arrow), which we'll discuss next.

10   **10**

The parietal pleura is somewhat adherent to the internal surface of the chest wall and is not readily
stripped away. For this reason the superior and
inferior edges of an extrapleural lesion usually are
tapered. This tapering and the _____ _____
contour are 2 of the signs that mark the extrapleural lesion.   sharp

11   **11**

The upper and lower edges of an extrapleural lesion   tapered
usually are _____. The margin is _____.   sharp

Figure 8-2 illustrates an extrapleural hematoma secondary to recent
chest trauma. The margin facing the lung is sharp and the superior
border is tapered.

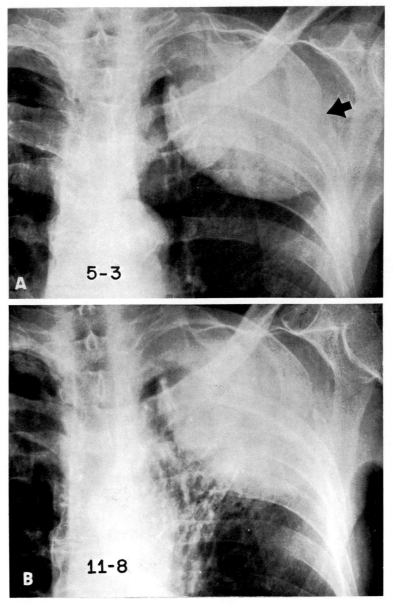

Figure 8-3

12

You may have noted in Figures 8-1 and 8-2 that the extrapleural lesions were convex toward the lung. This convexity is a third roentgen sign of extrapleural disease. What are the other 2 signs again?

(1) _____ _____
(2) _____ _____

12

(1) sharp border

(2) tapering edges

13

A fourth sign is related to the commonest source of extrapleural disease, _____ destruction.

13

rib

14

Extrapleural lesions *usually* do not break into the pleural space. Therefore pleural thickening and pleural effusion generally are (present / absent) with extrapleural lesions.

14

absent

15

If extension through the parietal pleura does occur, most of the extrapleural signs disappear. But one sign, if it was present originally, always remains. Which? _____ _____

15

rib destruction

Figure 8-3 illustrates extension of metastatic extrapleural tumor through the pleura and into the lung. All the extrapleural signs in A, except the rib destruction (arrow), have disappeared in B, which was obtained 6 months later.

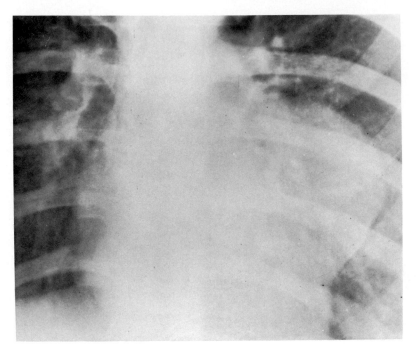

Figure 8–4

16

List at least 4 roentgen signs of extrapleural lesions:

(1) ** _____
(2) ** _____
(3) ** _____
(4) ** _____
(5) ** _____

16

(1) sharp border

(2) tapering margins

(3) convexity toward lung

(4) rib destruction

(5) absence of pleural involvement

17

Not every extrapleural lesion exhibits all these changes, nor are the individual signs pathognomonic, except for (rib / lung) involvement.

17

rib

18

Encapsulated pleural fluid may closely simulate an extrapleural lesion. If pleural thickening is present elsewhere in the affected hemithorax, the lesion is probably (pleural / extrapleural).

18

pleural

19

The mediastinum is, in effect, extrapleural. It lies just outside both pleural cavities, doesn't it?

Which one of the extrapleural signs obviously *cannot* apply to an extrapleural mediastinal mass bulging into the lung? _____ _____

19

rib involvement

Figure 8-4 illustrates a mediastinal dermoid tumor. Note the convexity, sharp margin, and tapering inferior edge.

REVIEW

List the 5 extrapleural signs and circle the one that does not apply to a mediastinal mass. If you don't get them all, you have earned the award of the constipated termite.*

(1) ** _____
(2) ** _____
(3) ** _____
(4) ** _____
(5) ** _____

(1) sharp border

(2) tapering edges

(3) convexity toward lung

(4) rib destruction

(5) absence of pleural involvement

* He couldn't pass his boards.

Chapter 9

THE MANY CAUSES OF RIB NOTCHING

We offer this chapter as a bonus. While it doesn't quite mesh with the subject matter of the rest of the book, it is important and does embody certain principles of chest roentgenology. Besides, it was available.*

1

How many causes of rib notching do you know? Write them down:

1

You probably wrote *coarctation of the aorta* and then were stuck. That's by far the commonest, but there are many others.

2

Notching of the inferior margin of a rib is generally caused by enlargement of one of 3 important structures in the intercostal space: the _____, the vein, or the nerve.

2

artery

* This chapter is based on an exhibit by M. L. Boone, B. E. Swenson, B. Felson, H. B. Spitz, and A. S. Weinstein, shown in 1963 at the American Roentgen Ray Society meeting in Montreal and at the Radiological Society of North America meeting in Chicago. Most of the illustrations were taken, with permission, from an article of the same title by M. L. Boone, B. E. Swenson, and B. Felson, published in Am. J. Roentgenol., *91:* 1075, 1964 (Charles C Thomas, Springfield, Illinois).

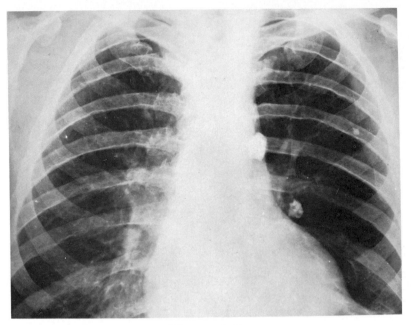

Figure 9-1

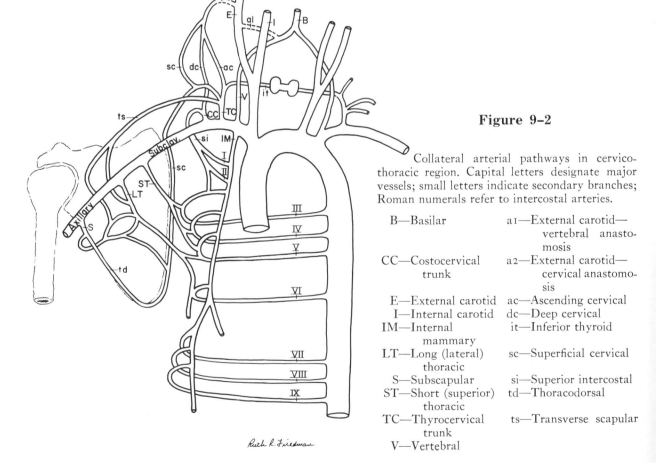

Figure 9-2

Collateral arterial pathways in cervico-thoracic region. Capital letters designate major vessels; small letters indicate secondary branches; Roman numerals refer to intercostal arteries.

B—Basilar	a1—External carotid— vertebral anastomosis
CC—Costocervical trunk	a2—External carotid— cervical anastomosis
E—External carotid	ac—Ascending cervical
I—Internal carotid	dc—Deep cervical
IM—Internal mammary	it—Inferior thyroid
LT—Long (lateral) thoracic	sc—Superficial cervical
S—Subscapular	si—Superior intercostal
ST—Short (superior) thoracic	td—Thoracodorsal
TC—Thyrocervical trunk	ts—Transverse scapular
V—Vertebral	

3   **3**

First, let's discuss the intercostal arteries. Certainly,
the best known and commonest cause of rib notch-   coarctation
ing is _____ of the _____.
In this condition notching is caused by the dilated   aorta
and tortuous _____ arteries.
                                                          intercostal

Note the rib notching in Figure 9-1. This 72 year old asymptomatic man
has coarctation of the aorta. Longevity is unusual in coarctation.
Incidentally, the terms *scalloping* (shallow wave-like indentations) and
notching (narrow deep indentations) are used interchangeably since
these deformities have the same significance.

4   **4**

In coarctation, blood must bypass the aortic con-
striction to get to the abdomen and lower extremities.
The collateral pathways arise almost exclusively from
the 2 subclavian arteries. The blood then passes
via the thyrocervical, costocervical, and internal
_____ branches of the subclavian, and the
subdivisions of these arteries, to reach the posterior   mammary
intercostals. The blood in these intercostals then
flows (toward / away from) the descending aorta.   toward

Trace the collateral flow from the subclavian to the posterior intercostal
arteries in Figure 9-2.

5   **5**

Let's review this again by means of an arterial flow chart:

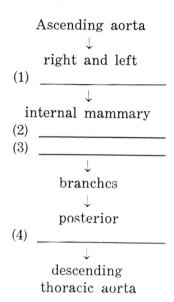

Ascending aorta
↓
right and left
(1) _____
↓
internal mammary
(2) _____
(3) _____
↓
branches
↓
posterior
(4) _____
↓
descending
thoracic aorta

(1) subclavians

(2) thyrocervical

(3) costocervical

(4) intercostals

"The flow of fluids is always from the higher pressure to the lower pressure area."*

---

6   **6**

In coarctation the notching usually involves several posterior ribs bilaterally, from the 3rd through the 9th. The first 2 intercostal arteries do not connect directly to the _____ and the last 3 have no connection to the subclavian system (see Figure 9-2 again).

aorta

The *anterior* intercostals, arising from the internal mammaries, are paired in each intercostal space. They do not lie close to the anterior ribs and therefore do not notch them.

---

* Tu Hunghai: Chinese Med. J., *14:* 281, 1372 B.C.

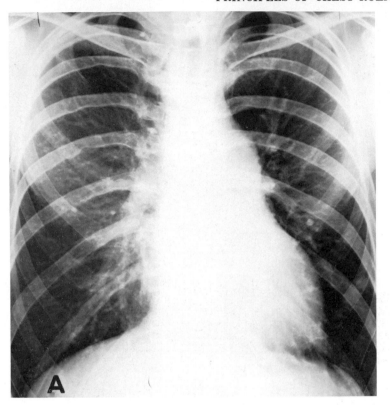

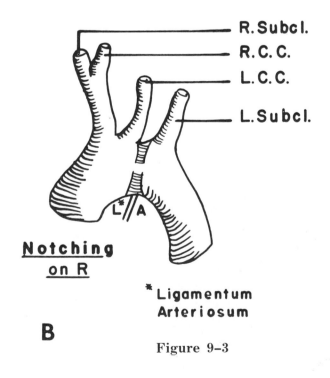

Figure 9–3

7   7

If the coarctation lies distal to the left subclavian
artery, as it almost always does, the notching will
be bilateral. If the coarctation lies proximal to the
left subclavian artery, the rib notching will be
(unilateral / bilateral).   unilateral

The high pressure in the subclavian arteries in coarctation favors the
filling of collateral pathways. When the *left* subclavian arises distal to
the coarctation (Figure 9-3, *B*), the pressure in this artery is low, and
notching will only be present on the *right* (Figure 9-3, *A*). The notching in this patient is confined to the right 5th to 7th ribs.*

* Courtesy Dr. John A. Campbell, Indianapolis.

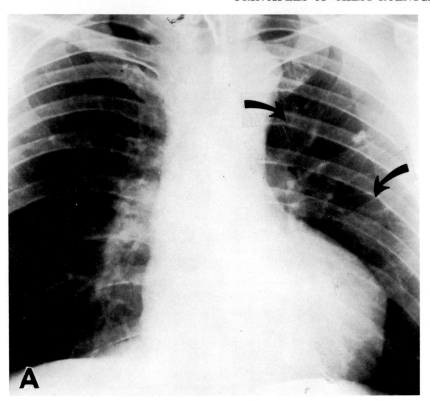

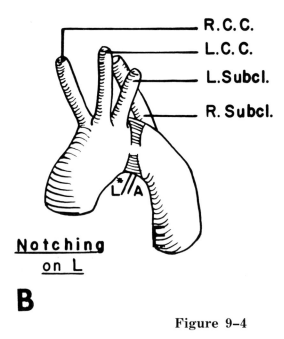

Figure 9-4

8   8

If there is an *anomalous* right subclavian artery
that arises distal to the coarctation, the notching
will be unilateral. Since little blood is reaching the
right subclavian artery, the pressure in this artery
is too low to permit collateral flow, and the notching will be confined to the _____
side.   left

> Figure 9-4 is an example of this. The left 6th and 7th ribs are notched
> (arrows).*

9   9

Thus, unilateral rib notching can occur in coarctation, and one can then usually predict the pathologic
anatomy of the aortic arch. The notching is always
on the (same / opposite) side as the subclavian
artery which comes off proximal to the coarctation.   same

10   10

O.K., let's summarize coarctation. The collateral flow
is:

Aorta
↓
right and left
(1) _____
↓
(2) _____
(3) _____
(4) _____
↓
their branches
↓
posterior
(5) _____
↓
descending
thoracic aorta

(1) subclavian

(2) internal mammary

(3) thyrocervical

(4) costocervical

(5) intercostals

* Courtesy Dr. John A. Campbell, Indianapolis.

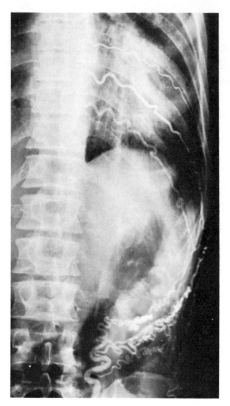

Figure 9-5

11

Rib notching involves the _____ through the _____ ribs. Are all these ribs notched in an individual patient? (Usually / Seldom)

11

3rd

9th

Seldom

12

More summarizing and then we're through with this. Notching confined to the right ribs usually indicates that the _____ subclavian artery arises distal to the coarctation. Notching confined to the left side usually indicates that the _____ subclavian artery comes off distal to the coarctation.

12

left

right

Now let's really get down to work.

13

In thrombosis of the abdominal aorta, the lower intercostal arteries serve as collaterals to the lower part of the body. They become large and tortuous and may cause notching of the lower ribs. Obviously, here the intercostal artery flow is (toward / away from) the aorta.

13

away from

In Figure 9-5 the thoracic aortogram shows abdominal aortic occlusion with dilatation of the 8th to 10th intercostal arteries, which carry blood to the lower part of the body. Note the tortuous lower intercostals indenting the ribs.

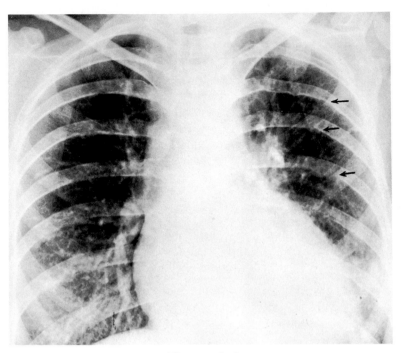

Figure 9–6

14   14

You have now learned 2 mechanisms and 2 causes
of rib notching.

Mechanism

(a) High aortic obstruction. (Intercostal flow is
_____ the aorta.)

(b) Low aortic obstruction. (Intercostal flow is
_____ the aorta.)

Cause

(1) Coarctation of aorta   toward

(2) Thrombosis of abdominal aorta   from

15   15

Deficient blood flow to the arm occurs following the
Blalock-Taussig (subclavian-pulmonary artery) anas-
tomosis for tetralogy of Fallot. A good part of
the arterial collateral flow to the arm is:

Aorta

↓

posterior
intercostals

↓

long and short
thoracics

↓

axillary

This may eventually result in (unilateral / bilateral)   unilateral (on the same
rib notching.   side as the operation)

Figure 9-6 shows a child with notching of the 3rd to 7th left ribs (arrows) which appeared after a left Blalock-Taussig operation.

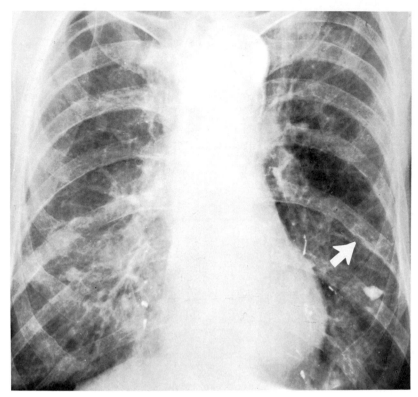

Figure 9–7

16

"Pulseless disease" is caused by either arteritis (Takayasu's disease) or arteriosclerosis obliterans. It is associated with occlusion of 2 or more of the brachiocephalic arteries at their origin. This results in diminished flow to the _____, similar to that following the _____ _____ operation, and the collateral flow is much the same. So here is another arterial cause of rib notching.

arm

Blalock-Taussig

Figure 9-7 is an example of pulseless disease from severe arteriosclerosis of all the great vessels arising from the aortic arch. The left 8th rib shows definite notching (arrow).

17

Following the Blalock-Taussig procedure and in pulseless disease, the blood flow in the intercostal arteries is (toward / away from) the aorta. In these 2 conditions the rib notching will be on the (side of / side opposite) the occluded subclavian artery.

away from

side of

18

You should now know 4 arterial causes of rib notching. Do you?

High aortic obstruction: (1) _____

Low aortic obstruction: (2) _____

Subclavian obstruction: (3) _____

(4) pulseless disease

(1) coarctation

(2) aortic thrombosis

(3) Blalock-Taussig operation

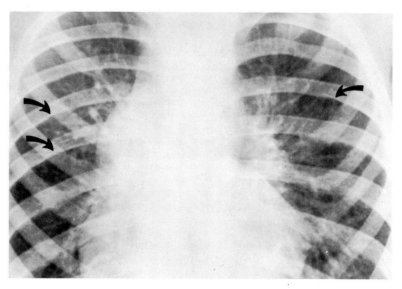

Figure 9–8

19

Next we have several conditions which occasionally cause arterial rib notching by another mechanism. In congenital cardiovascular lesions with decreased pulmonary blood flow, the pulmonary circulation may be augmented by blood from the intercostal arteries via the bronchial arteries, branches perforating through the chest wall, etc. Example: tetralogy of Fallot.

Can you think of some other congenital lesions with decreased pulmonary flow?

(1) __ ** _____
(2) __ ** _____
(3) __ ** _____

19

(1) pulmonary valvular stenosis

(2) absent pulmonary artery

(3) pseudotruncus (atresia of the main pulmonary artery)

Figure 9-8: tetralogy of Fallot with absent right pulmonary artery. The notching of the left 6th rib (arrow) appeared a year after the Blalock-Taussig operation. The notching on the right (arrows) antedated the operation. So there are 2 mechanisms for rib notching in this patient.

20

Four congenital cardiovascular lesions with decreased pulmonary flow in which rib notching has been reported are:

(1) pseudotruncus
(2) _____ pulmonary artery
(3) _____ of _____
(4) _____ valvular stenosis

20

(2) absent

(3) tetralogy of Fallot

(4) pulmonary

Curiously, all the cases so far reported have had unilateral notching. Don't ask us why.

Whoops — we just saw a report in which *pulmonary emphysema* resulted in rib notching by this same mechanism, i.e., decreased pulmonary circulation with intercostal arteries supplying the oligemic lung. We've got an example, but didn't realize it — had it labeled "idiopathic."

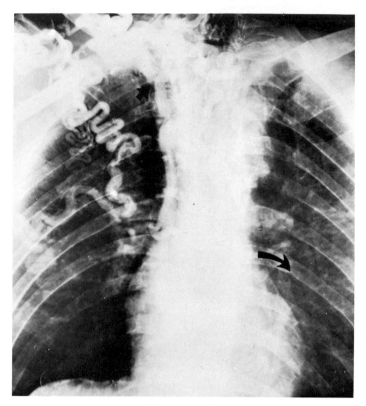

Figure 9–9

21

O.K., here are 4 mechanisms and 9 causes of *arterial* rib notching:

(a) _____
   (1) _____
(b) low aortic obstruction:
   (2) _____
(c) subclavian obstruction:
   (3) _____
   (4) _____
(d) pulmonary oligemia:
   (5) _____
   (6) _____
   (7) _____
   (8) _____
   (9) _____

21

(a) high aortic obstruction

(1) coarctation of aorta
(2) aortic thrombosis
(3) Blalock-Taussig procedure
(4) pulseless disease
(5) tetralogy of Fallot
(6) absent pulmonary artery
(7) pulmonary valvular stenosis
(8) pseudotruncus
(9) emphysema

22

Now what about the intercostal veins. Can they cause notching? Sure — or else we wouldn't have brought it up.

Fibrosing mediastinitis may cause chronic obstruction of the _____ vena cava. The azygos system becomes a major collateral pathway, and the intercostal veins often carry a considerable amount of blood to the _____ system.

22

superior

azygos

23

The intercostal veins may become so dilated and tortuous that they notch the ribs. So far, the only reported cause of venous notching has been obstruction of the ** _____ secondary to _____ _____.

23

superior vena cava

fibrosing mediastinitis

Figure 9-9 is a right brachial venogram showing superior vena cava obstruction and numerous collateral veins in the neck and mediastinum. A large tortuous intercostal vein is notching the right 5th rib. The left 8th rib is also notched (arrow).

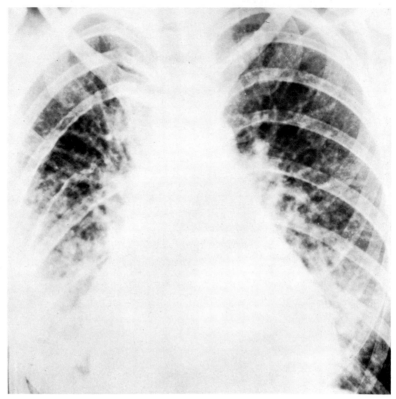

Figure 9–10

24   24

Arteriovenous fistulas are characterized by large
feeding and draining vessels. The intercostal vessels
may be involved and notch the ribs. Can you name
2 sites of an arteriovenous fistula in which this
might occur?

                                     (1) chest wall

   (1) ** _____

   (2) ** _____   (2) pulmonary

> Notching caused by arteriovenous fistula is the one most people forget.
> Will you?
>   Figure 9-10 shows innumerable tiny pulmonary arteriovenous fistulas
> in a patient with congenital familial telangiectases.* The right 5th
> and 7th ribs show notching (the 6th has been resected).

25   25

You have now learned an even dozen causes of rib   arteriovenous
notching — 9 arterial, 1 venous, and 2 _____.
  Fill in the appropriate responses: (a) high aortic obstruc-
          I. Arterial   tion
  (a) _____ (1) _____   (b) low aortic obstruc-
  (b) _____ (2) _____   tion
  (c) subclavian obstruction (3) _____   (d) pulmonary oligemia
                  (4) _____
  (d) _____ (5) _____   (1) coarctation of aorta
                  (6) _____   (2) aortic thrombosis
                  (7) _____   (3) Blalock-Taussig
                  (8) _____   procedure
                  (9) _____   (4) pulseless disease
          II. Venous   (5) tetralogy of Fallot
               (10) _____   (6) absent pulmonary
     III. Arteriovenous   artery
               (11) _____   (7) pulmonary valvular
               (12) _____   stenosis
                                          (8) pseudotruncus
                                          (9) emphysema
                                          (10) superior vena cava
                                              obstruction
                                          (11) A-V fistula of chest
                                          wall
                                          (12) pulmonary A-V
                                          fistula

* Courtesy Dr. Russell H. Morgan, Baltimore.

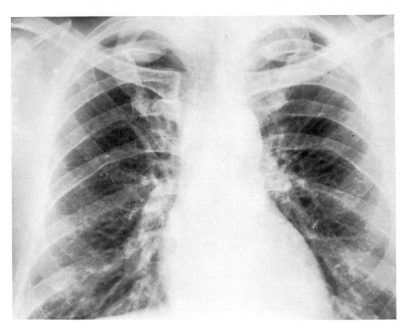

Figure 9–11

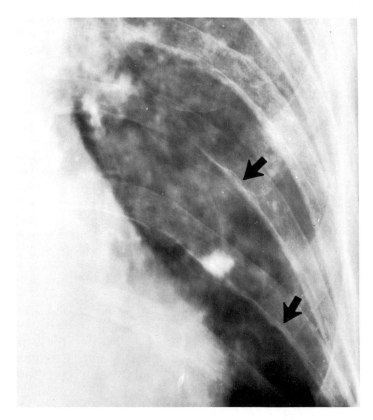

Figure 9–12

26   **26**

The third important component of the intercostal
space is the _____. If there is a
tumor of this structure, rib notching may occur.   nerve

In neurofibromatosis, these notches may be multiple.
Figure 9-11 shows notching of the right 4th to 7th and left 6th to 8th
ribs in a patient with neurofibromatosis. The mass in each pulmonary
apex represents an intercostal neuroma.

27   **27**

Thus, rib notching may be caused by artery, vein,
or _____ lesions. Rarely, the cause
of the notching cannot be determined. So we must
include an idiopathic category.* We have seen one
such case with striking notches in many ribs.   nerve

28   **28**

One of the authors (B.F.) reviewed 1000 normal
survey chest roentgenograms for rib notching, and
encountered it in mild degree (never severe) in 1 or
2 ribs with surprising frequency. (He probably has
a _____ retina.)   notched

Figure 9-12 shows these "normal" rib indentations (arrows) simulating
notching or scalloping. You may have noted in some of the earlier
illustrations that the notches were rather minimal in degree. Obviously,
the recognition of *bona fide* notching is not always easy.

29   **29**

So here are 3 more causes of rib notching:

IV. nerve   (13) _____
V. idiopathic   (14) idiopathic
VI. normal!   (15) normal   (13) neurofibromatosis

* Idio — I don't know; pathic — I wish I did.

REVIEW

You have learned 15 causes of rib notching. We admit there may be others but, if so, they're about as common as priapism in the old men's home. Classify the ones you know in the space below:

Mechanism

I. _____   (a) _____   (1) _____

                        (b) _____   (2) _____

                        (c) _____   (3) _____

                                                  (4) _____

                        (d) _____   (5) _____

                                                  (6) _____

                                                  (7) _____

                                                  (8) _____

                                                  (9) _____

II. _____   (10) _____

III. _____   (11) _____

                                                  (12) _____

IV. _____   (13) _____

V. _____   (14) _____

VI. _____   (15) _____

I. Arterial   (a) high aortic obstruction   (1) coarctation of aorta
                   (b) low aortic obstruction   (2) aortic thrombosis
                   (c) subclavian obstruction   (3) Blalock-Taussig
                                                procedure
                                          (4) pulseless disease

                   (d) pulmonary oligemia   (5) tetralogy of Fallot
                                          (6) absent pulmonary
                                                artery
                                         (7) pulmonary valvular
                                                stenosis
                                          (8) pseudotruncus
                                          (9) emphysema

II. Venous   (10) superior vena cava
                                              obstruction

III. Arteriovenous   (11) A-V fistula of chest
                                                wall
                                          (12) pulmonary A-V fistula

IV. Nerve   (13) neurofibromatosis
 V. Idiopathic   (14) idiopathic
VI. Normal   (15) normal

Now compare your answer to the one you gave in Frame 1.

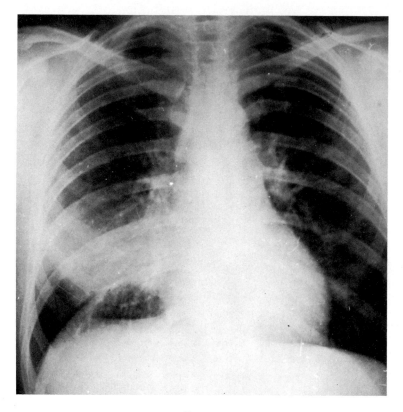

Case 1

This chapter consists of 10 cases presented to test your ability to apply the fundamental principles you have learned. We suggest that you answer all the questions on a case before turning the page to check the answers.

Case 1

This acutely ill young man has pneumonia.

1. In what lobe? _____

2. Why did you localize it to that lobe?
   ** _____

3. Name 2 views that would help you confirm your localization:
   ** _____

4. Name and number the involved segments:
   ** _____
   ** _____

Case 1

1. RML

2. Silhouette sign — the right heart border is obliterated.
   (See Chapter 4, Frame 17.)

3. Right lateral and lordotic views
   (See Chapter 1, Frame 22.)

4. #4 Lateral segment
   #5 Medial segment
   (See Chapter 3, Frames 8 and 9.)

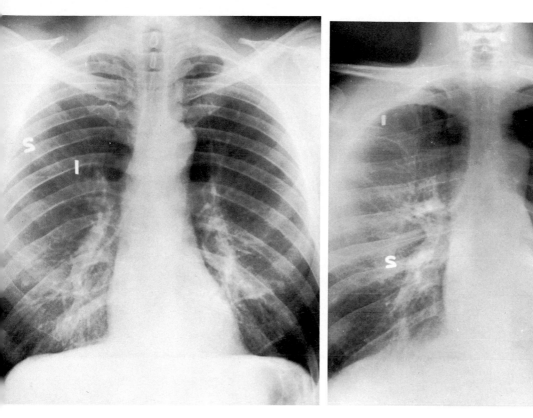

A   B

Case 2

1. In this healthy patient, Figure *A* is, of course, a PA teleo. What view is shown in *B*?

   **
   _____

2. The lead letters are taped to the chest wall. No. 1 is on the (anterior / posterior) chest wall and No. 2 is on the (anterior / posterior) chest wall.

   Suggestion: Place your finger in the suspected position of No. 1 in *A*. Now assume the position illustrated in *B*. Do the same for No. 2.
   Another suggestion: Don't do this in public — they'll take you away.

3. What are the 2 main indications for the view shown in *B*?

   **
   _____

   **
   _____

Case 2

1. Lordotic view (Note the elevated clavicles and horizontal position of the ribs.)

2. No. 1 is anterior; No. 2 is posterior

3. For better delineation of apical lesions
   For better demonstration of RML or lingular disease
   (See Chapter 1, Frames 21 and 22.)

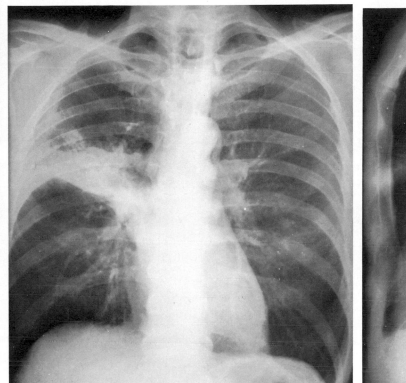 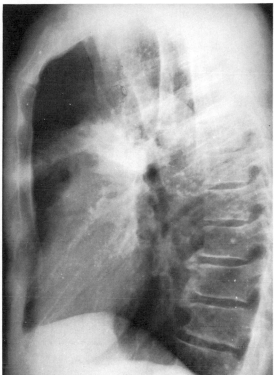

A   B

Case 3

This is a chronically ill 55 year old man.

1. On the PA teleo (Figure *A*), what structure is obliterated by the obvious lesion?

    ** _____

2. What is responsible for the sharp inferior margin of the lesion?

    ** _____

3. Name and number the segment involved:

    ** _____

4. Do you think that collapse of this segment is present? Why?

    ** _____

Case 3

1. Ascending aorta

2. Minor fissure (See Chapter 2, Frame 14.)

3. #2, anterior segment of the RUL (See Chapter 4, Frame 18.)

4. Yes. There is upward displacement of the minor fissure.
    (See Chapter 6, Frame 41.)

The patient had a bronchogenic carcinoma of the anterior segment bronchus of the RUL with central obstruction collapse.

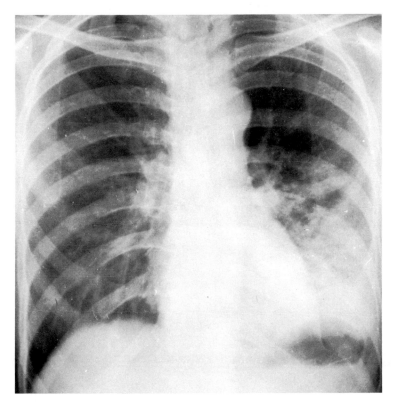

Case 4

This patient has obvious disease in the left lower thorax.

1. What structure does it obliterate?
    **

2. What structure does it fail to obliterate?
    **

3. What is the position of the left hilum compared to the right?
    **

4. What is the x-ray diagnosis?
    **

Case 4

1. Left hemidiaphragm (See Chapter 4, Frame 39.)

2. Left heart border

3. Lower

4. LLL collapse (See Chapter 6, Frames 21, 22, and 24.)

The patient had pneumonia with peripherial obstruction collapse.

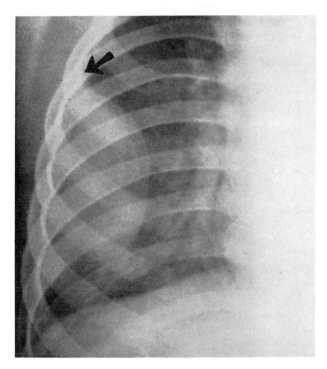

Case 5

Here is an asymptomatic patient with an interesting chest lesion.

1. In what anatomic location is the lesion?

    ** _____

2. What characteristic feature of this type of lesion is pointed out by the arrow?

    ** _____

3. Name 2 other signs of this particular type of lesion shown by the patient:

    ** _____

4. Which sign of such lesions is absent in this patient?

    ** _____

5. List some categories of diseases which produce this type of lesion:

    ** _____

Case 5

1. Extrapleural (chest wall)

2. Tapering edge (See Chapter 8, Frame 10.)

3. Sharp border
    Convexity toward lung
    Absence of pleural involvement
    (See Chapter 8, Frames 9, 12, and 14.)

4. Rib destruction

5. Neoplasm, especially rib metastasis
    Infection
    Hematoma
    (See Chapter 8, Frame 7.)

    This was a lipoma.

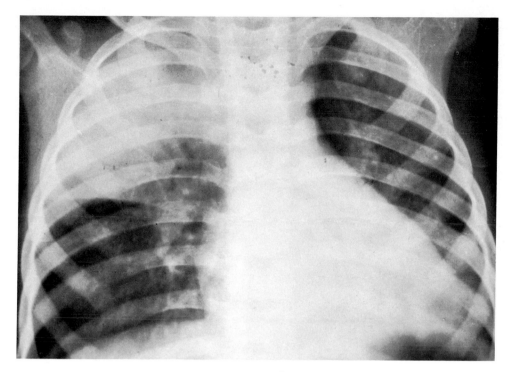

Case 6

This child has obvious pneumonia.

1. In what lobe?
    **
    _____

2. What structure is responsible for the sharp lower border?
    **
    _____

3. What structure is obviously obliterated by this pneumonia?
    **
    _____

    This indicates that at least segment #2 is involved. Name this segment:
    **
    _____

4. Look closely at the left thorax. What abnormalities do you see?
    **
    _____

    In what lobe do they indicate involvement?
    **
    _____

Case 6

1. RUL

2. Minor fissure (See Chapter 2, Frame 14.)

3. Ascending aorta
   Anterior segment of RUL

4. Obliteration of the left hemidiaphragm and air bronchogram; there is also an air bronchogram in the RUL. Subtle findings, aren't they?
   LLL

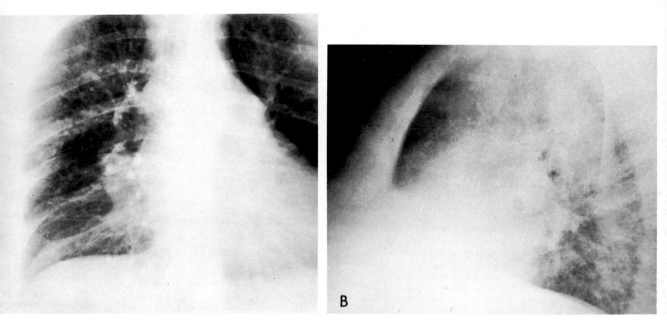

Case 7

This markedly obese woman had these routine films taken as part of a physical examination.

1. What sign of disease do you see on the PA teleo view (Figure *A*)?
    **
    _____

2. This sign indicates a lesion (anteriorly / posteriorly) even though you can't see the lesion itself.

3. Now that you know where to look on the lateral view, do you see the lesion?

    _____

4. What view would you order to see the lesion best?
    **
    _____

Case 7

1. Silhouette sign (The right heart border is obliterated.)

2. Anteriorly

3. No. The patient is so obese that the routine lateral view does not penetrate the lesion. The breasts also obscure it.

4. Bucky right lateral view (Figure C). The arrows point to a large antero-inferior mediastinal mass. Compare this with the routine lateral view in Figure B. (See Chapter 1, Frame 34.)

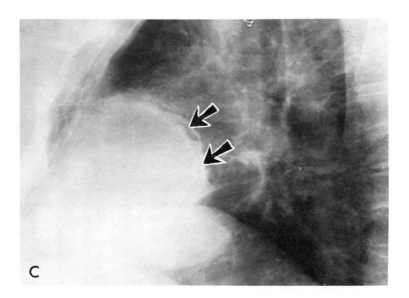

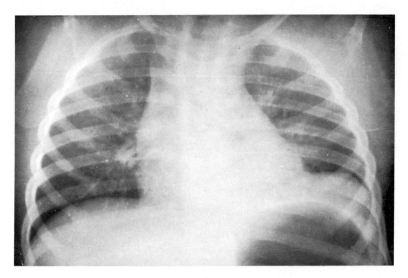

Λ

Case 8

Television is bad for kids! This 20 month old infant fell on a television antenna, which penetrated the chest.

1. Which pleural cavity was penetrated? _____ How do you know?

   ✳✳ _____

2. What view would you order to confirm it?

   ✳✳ _____

3. What other roentgen pattern does this condition sometimes show?

   ✳✳ _____

Case 8

1. Left. There is subpulmonary pleural effusion. We presume that you noted the elevation of the left "hemidiaphragm" and its separation from the gastric bubble.

2. Left lateral decubitus view (Figure *B*). (See Chapter 1, Frames 14 and 15.)

3. Meniscus pattern (See Chapter 7, Frame 7.)

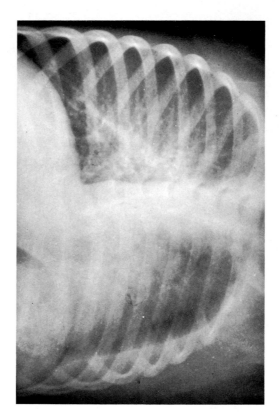

B

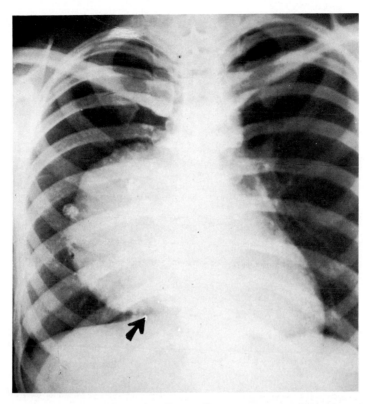

Case 9

1. Does this large mass lie in the lung or in the mediastinum?   Justify your answer.

    ** _____

2. The arrow points to the inferior edge of the right heart border. Does the mass lie anteriorly or posteriorly? _____ Justify your answer.

    ** _____

Case 9

1. Mediastinum. There are extrapleural signs: sharp lateral border, tapering edge, convex margin.

2. Anteriorly. The right heart border and ascending aorta are obliterated.

   The lesion proved to be a lymphoma of the anterior mediastinal lymph nodes.

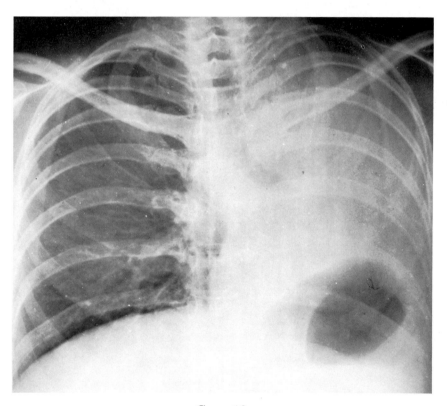

Case 10

Case 10

This is a chronically ill, heavy-smoking 60 year old man. With an assist from us, you should be able to localize the lesion and maybe even make the diagnosis.

1. Where is the heart?

    ** _____

2. Is the position of the gas bubble of the stomach normal? _____

3. Can you actually see the top of the left hemidiaphragm? _____
    Localize the disease in the vicinity of the left hemidiaphragm:

    ** _____

4. Can you see the descending thoracic aorta? _____
    Localize the disease in the vicinity of the descending thoracic aorta:

    ** _____

5. Can you see the left heart border? _____
    Localize the disease in the vicinity of the left heart border:

    ** _____

6. Can you see the aortic knob? _____
    Localize the disease in the vicinity of the aortic knob:

    ** _____

7. Add up the involved segments. What is the total?

    ** _____

8. After noting the position of the heart and left hemidiaphragm, and the appearance of the left main bronchus, what do you think is the likely diagnosis?

    ** _____

Case 10

1. Shifted into the left hemithorax
   (See Chapter 6, Frame 28.)

2. No. It is elevated.

3. No. Basal segments, LLL   =   # 7, 8, 9, 10

4. No. Superior and posterior segments, LLL   =   #6, 10
   (See Chapter 4, Frames 36 and 37.)

5. No. Anterior segment and lingula, LUL   =   #2, 4, 5
   (See Chapter 4, Frames 21 to 24.)

6. No. Apical-posterior segment, LUL   =   _____#1-3_____
   (See Chapter 4, Frames 27 to 29.)

7. #1-3 + 2, 4, 5 + 6 + 7, 8, 9, 10   = entire left lung
   This is the new mathematics.

8. Diagnosis: collapse from bronchogenic carcinoma in the left main bronchus.

INDEX

Pages with even numbers refer to illustrations.